Palgrave Studies in Animals and Literature

Various academic disciplines can now be found in the process of executing an 'animal turn', questioning the ethical and philosophical grounds of human exceptionalism by taking seriously the nonhuman animal presences that haunt the margins of history, anthropology, philosophy, sociology and literary studies. Such work is characterised by a series of broad, cross-disciplinary questions. How might we rethink and problematise the separation of the human from other animals? What are the ethical and political stakes of our relationships with other species? How might we locate and understand the agency of animals in human cultures?

This series publishes work that looks, specifically, at the implications of the 'animal turn' for the field of English Studies. Language is often thought of as the key marker of humanity's difference from other species; animals may have codes, calls or songs, but humans have a mode of communication of a wholly other order. The primary motivation is to muddy this assumption and to animalise the canons of English Literature by rethinking representations of animals and interspecies encounter. Whereas animals are conventionally read as objects of fable, allegory or metaphor (and as signs of specifically human concerns), this series significantly extends the new insights of interdisciplinary animal studies by tracing the engagement of such figuration with the material lives of animals. It examines textual cultures as variously embodying a debt to or an intimacy with animals and advances understanding of how the aesthetic engagements of literary arts have always done more than simply illustrate natural history. We publish studies of the representation of animals in literary texts from the Middle Ages to the present and with reference to the discipline's key thematic concerns, genres and critical methods. The series focuses on literary prose and poetry, while also accommodating related discussion of the full range of materials and texts and contexts (from theatre and film to fine art, journalism, the law, popular writing and other cultural ephemera) with which English studies now engages.

Lucinda Cole

The Fifth Plague

Cattle, Contagion, and the Medical Posthumanities

palgrave
macmillan

Lucinda Cole
University of Illinois Urbana-Champaign
Champaign, IL, USA

ISSN 2634-6338 ISSN 2634-6346 (electronic)
Palgrave Studies in Animals and Literature
ISBN 978-3-031-92792-8 ISBN 978-3-031-92793-5 (eBook)
https://doi.org/10.1007/978-3-031-92793-5

This Palgrave Macmillan imprint is published by the registered company Springer Nature Switzerland AG.
The registered company address is: Gewerbestrasse 11, 6330 Cham, Switzerland

For the healers and the fighters
Jean Cole, Ana Castro, Sonja Bjelić, Hannah Markley,
and Marcella, the little warrior

Acknowledgments

This book is indebted to countless animal studies scholars whose work has shaped my own over the past two decades. Susan McHugh helped to create the field of animal studies, both as brilliant scholar and as generous editor. *The Fifth Plague* owes its timely publication to her, to Robert McKay, and to John Miller, along with Linda Braus and the editorial team at Palgrave Macmillan. Anita Guerrini remains my often-unacknowledged scholarly north star.

Many thanks to the journals and presses who have allowed me to reprint sections of previously published essays. Part of Chapter 2 appeared as "Out of Africa: Infestation, Universal History, and the Early Modern Theological Imaginary" in a monumental two-volume collection on insects—*Lesser Creatures of the Renaissance*—edited by Keith Botelho and Joseph Campana, and published in 2023 by Pennsylvania State University Press. Chapter 3 began several years ago as an essay in the *Routledge Handbook of Shakespeare and Animals*, edited by Karen Raber and Holly Dugan. Chapter 4, on Daniel Defoe, originated in a plenary lecture at the Society for Eighteenth-Century Studies/Société canadienne d'étude du dix-huitième siècle (CSECS/SCEDHS), later published in *Lumen*. The final chapter, on cholera and the 1865–67 outbreaks, grew out of an international conference whose papers appeared in *Animals and Epidemics: Interspecies Entanglements in Historical Perspective*, edited by Mieke Roscher, Axel Hüntelmann, Christian Jaser, and Nadir Weber.

Colleagues at the University of Illinois have supported this project throughout its many stages. Jane Desmond and Jamie Jones, of the Animal

Turn Research Cluster Group, brought me in and gave me an institutional home. Gillen D'arcy Wood welcomed me to the Institute for Sustainability, Energy, and the Environment, from which I learn something new every day. Melissa Littlefield, Curtis Perry, Tony Pollock, Robert Parker, Justine Murison, Clare Crowston—all have stepped in or stepped up at key moments. I am forever grateful. Dana Smith, the perfect research assistant, took time from her graduate studies to help with both scholarship and editing. Michael Knierim accepted the challenge of translating a tricky Latin poem which, as it turned out, helped structure this book.

Even closer to home are members of my writing group. Melissa Mowry, Dana Rabin, and Andrea McKenzie keep me on track and more or less sane while the world shakes. I am lucky to know them. Stephen Markley, similarly, offers a lovable model of how to work, laugh, and meet deadlines. It is impossible to imagine contemporary life without Pat Gill, Richard Wheeler, Bret Tonelli, Rick Barney, Ramón Soto-Crespo, and Tim Dean, all of whom are at the ready with encouragement and reality checks. Melanie—you're in my heart. Hunter Cole Matthews and Richard Abrams passed away, suddenly, while this book was in press. I wish I could have told them goodbye, and thank you. As for Robert Markley, it has been a tough few years, with one plague following another. Without Bob, both this book and I would probably be in pieces on the floor.

Competing Interests The author has no competing interests to declare that are relevant to the content of this manuscript.

Contents

List of Figures

CHAPTER 1

Cattle, Disease, and the Stories We Tell

Abstract Serving as an introduction to *The Fifth Plague: Cattle, Contagion, and the Medical Posthumanities*, this chapter argues for a strategic alliance between the One Health movement, which attends to cross-species epidemics, and the health humanities, which tend to focus on humans alone. I call this approach the medical posthumanities. *The Fifth Plague* contributes to the medical posthumanities in a specific way: it offers a transdisciplinary history of cattle plagues and their real or imagined cross-species contagions, thereby illuminating the shared vulnerability of humans and livestock in global cattle-grain regimes. That causal explanations for repeated and devastating cattle plagues are rarely unyoked from both classical and Christian disease ecologies make this kind of cross-disciplinary reading necessary for understanding the past, and helpful for appreciating the present; zoonotic diseases circulate around and through us at an alarming rate, their causes and cures still tethered in many ways to Christian scourge logic.

Now of diseases, what the Law, and whence
The Influences of bane upgathering can
Upon the race of men and herds of cattle
Kindle a devastation fraught with death
I will unfold.
Lucretius, *De Rerum Natura*

L. Cole, *The Fifth Plague*, Palgrave Studies in Animals and Literature, https://doi.org/10.1007/978-3-031-92793-5_1

After my first year of college as an Animal and Dairy Science major, I scored a summer job with the Kentucky State Veterinarian's Office. Because they stuck me in a windowless office with endless piles of unfiled reports, I begged to do field work. Assuring the Director that I knew how to drive a stick shift (I did not), the Director gave me two new assignments, both central to the Office's mission: to protect the health and welfare of Kentucky's livestock, poultry, and agricultural industries. On Mondays, I'd take the office van to the Post Office in Frankfort, pick up severed dog heads in (sometimes oozing) black boxes, and deliver them to the University of Kentucky Veterinary Diagnostic Lab in Lexington, where they would be tested for rabies. But in August, I hit the temporary job jackpot—I accompanied my immediate supervisor to the Kentucky State Fair, tasked with ensuring that show cattle had been vaccinated against brucellosis. And because this was the week that Elvis died, and because my supervisor retreated to her hotel room to manage her grief, I was allowed to roam. Daily, I visited the cattle barns, checking numbered papers for the right ticked boxes, then numbers on the papers against numbered ear tags or tattoos on the cattle. Free, mobile, and flush with petty bureaucratic authority, I rolled all around the West Pavilion, through yawning halls of pigs, beef cattle, goats and cows penned, tied, or dragged around in show rings, then beyond those halls into places my state-issued golf cart probably should not have been.

Later, with a PhD in literature, I used to tell this story at academic cocktail parties under the rubric of "My Worst Job Ever" to make people laugh. There is—or was—something funny about livestock for many literary people, a giggly discomfort that often shows up at eighteenth-century conferences when, in papers about the georgic, readers smirk at John Dyer's lines about "fairest flocks" rejoicing: "they, nor of halt,/ Hydropic tumors, nor of rot, complain;/ Evils deform'd and foul: nor with hoarse cough/ Disturb the music of the past'ral pipe" (Dyer 2019, ll. 20–24).[1] Anne Milne took full advantage of such cosmopolitan uneasiness in her book on eco-critical readings of animals and women in the poetry of Ann Yearsley and others, *Lactilla Tends Her Fav'rite Cow* (2008). Yet the "hoarse cough" that we do not hear in Dyer's *The Fleece* opens up literary studies to medical and environmental, as well as economic approaches; it signals our entangled relations with questions of animal health and their larger consequences for farmers, merchants, and consumers. Such a cough, according to Dyer's

[1] On the significance of *The Fleece* in eighteenth-century literary and imperial culture see Goodridge (1995, 91–98); Chico (2019, 101–121); and Menely (2021, 127–142). On agrarian literature in the seventeenth century see McRae (1996).

editors, John Goodridge and Juan Pellicer, can indicate either tuberculosis or brucellosis.[2] I did not know, when I was riding around at the fairgrounds, that brucellosis—also known as Malta fever, Mediterranean fever, or undulant fever—originates from an intracellular parasite, and that different strains of this disease can infect dogs, goats, sheep, pigs, and cattle. Brucellosis is one of forty-five common bovine pathogens—bacteria, viruses, fungi, parasites, and prions—capable of being transmitted zoonotically (McDaniel et al. 2014, 1–19). As a zoonotic disease, it can spread across species and cause fevers, arthritis, anemia, endocarditis, spontaneous abortion, and a host of neurological disorders. Although rarely fatal to those who have access to antibiotics, brucellosis can and has caused chronic diseases in populations that do not. Mussolini's doctor diagnosed a suffering William Butler Yeats with brucellosis in 1929 (Ross 2012, 147–166).

The Fifth Plague: Cattle, Contagion, and the Medical Posthumanities takes seriously the role of real and imagined diseases of cattle as historical agents within Judeo-Christian agrotheology. Set in Europe—especially Great Britain—my narrative is multispecies, ecological, and biopolitical; it includes sheep, cows, steer, oxen, insects, shepherds, husbandmen, farmers, physicians, poets, playwrights, theologians, historians, and, of course, governments. Like Timothy Morton, I treat epidemics as inevitable byproducts of "agrilogistics," a term Morton borrows to describe the gradual conversion of natural habitats into grazing pastures, thereby forcing animal populations, wild and domestic, into new and often dangerous proximities to humans, increasing the likelihood that evolving viruses will jump species, evolve again, and multiply zoonotic disease vectors (Morton 2016, 43). To a great extent, the history of mass mortality events—both human and animal—is the history of grain farming, and informing this book is a wide body of primary literature on animal husbandry and agricultural improvement. *The Fifth Plague* is also a history of plague bureaucracies. Agrilogistics gave rise to what Bruno Latour terms "centers of calculation" (Latour 1987, 245), concentrated populations where grain and livestock could be collected, counted, stored, and distributed; these centers of calculation with their bureaucratic technologies also functioned as centers of political and economic power with the authority to identify, record, and try to manage outbreaks of cattle disease. Between the sixteenth and nineteenth centuries, mitigation and containment policies led to millions of animals, either actually infected or merely exposed, being slaughtered in the names of public health and economic stability. The problems posed by cattle disease

[2] Goodridge and Pellicer, eds., *The Fleece*, note to line 12.

resonated throughout regions and nation-states, affecting the sociopolitical and agricultural health of regimes across Europe.

Scientists and physicians already have told parts of this story. In 2008, the American Veterinary Association cosponsored with the American Medical Association, the Center for Disease Control, environmental organizations, and other medical institutions the One Health Initiative. The AVMA's inaugural report on the One Health Initiative Task Force (2008) emphasizes that we are facing "demanding, profound, and unprecedented" challenges associated, in part, with a rising demand for "animal protein," a concomitant loss of biodiversity, and the increasing difficulty of containing the 75% of new, emergent human diseases that are zoonotic: "Our increasing interdependence with animals and their products may well be the single most critical risk factor" to human health.[3] Given the historical dependence of humans on cattle, a significant number of zoonotic diseases are spread either by agricultural workers on the front lines or by consuming meat, unpasteurized milk, and cheese from infected animals. Although India, Brazil, Europe, and the United States, followed closely by China, claim in the twenty-first century over half of the world's cattle population, perhaps surprisingly, zoonotic pathogens are distributed equally around the world. Authors of a recent review attribute this phenomenon to global transportation networks; long-distance movement of cattle from grazing sites, markets farms, feedlots, abattoirs, and grocery stores has allowed pathogens "to adapt to new environments and expand geographically" (McDaniel et al. 2014, 13). When it was founded, One Health thus understandably had as its visionary goal the creation of an epidemiological framework capable of addressing health problems so widespread and complex that no single nation, organization, or discipline could manage them. Abigail Woods and others have encouraged scientists to rethink the history of medicine as "a series of interspecies interactions" recognizing the role, past and present, that cattle play (Woods et al. 2018, 11). William H. McNeill insisted almost half a century ago that "most and probably all the distinctive infectious diseases of human civilization transferred to human civilizations from animal herds" (McNeill 1977, 445). This pattern continues, even as cattle populations explode. As of 2015, humans represented 34% of vertebrate biomass and vertebrate wildlife 4%.[4] The other 62% was composed of livestock, more than half of

[3] American Veterinary Medical Association (2008), accessed January 11, 2018. In later versions (accessed August 7, 2023), this statement was removed (King et al. 2008, 259–261).

[4] Morton (2016, 44). Morton's statistics differ slightly from those presented in Bar-On et al. (2018: 6506–6511).

that cattle, most of them pumped full of antibiotics in order to mitigate the effects of a monstrous agro-industrial machinery that, seemingly, we can neither quit nor live without.

After the BSE (Bovine spongiform encephalopathy, or "mad cow disease") breakouts in the mid-1980s, during which 4 million cattle were slaughtered to contain a disease that ended up killing nearly 200 persons, several important monographs and collections on cattle and disease appeared: Lise Wilkinson's *Animals and Disease: an Introduction to the History of Comparative Medicine* (1992); Clive Spinage's *Cattle Plague: A History* (2003); the edited collections *Healing the Herds: Disease, Livestock Economies, and the Globalization of Veterinary Medicine* (2010); and *Animals and the Shaping of Modern Medicine: One Health and Its Histories* (2018). Angela Cassidy's *Vermin, Victims, and Disease* (2019), similarly, focuses on the controversial question of culling badgers in order to control the spread of bovine tuberculosis in British cattle. In 2020, the global COVID-19 pandemic further jumpstarted humanist interest in zoonotic diseases, sometimes, but not always, in ways critical of anthropocentric blind spots.[5] For humanists, the most valuable of these recent collections is *Animals and Epidemics: Interspecies Entanglements in Historical Perspective* (2023), whose editors emphasize the role of animals as agents *both* in pandemics and in the stories we tell about them: "non-human actors emerge as potent co-actors in the shaping of epochs and their construction" (Hüntelmann et al. 2024, 11). From this historical perspective, which I share, stricken, quarantined, and sacrificed cattle become powerful actants in the economic, agricultural, medical, and cultural worlds of the sixteenth, seventeenth, eighteenth, and nineteenth centuries.

What *The Fifth Plague* contributes to this emerging field is an approach shaped by literary, historical, and epidemiological studies, but driven by animal studies. The medical humanities, grounded in work by Priscilla Wald (2008) and Melvin Santer (2014), among others, has been concerned for some time with epidemic disease and the problems of disease transmission. Wald, writing in the wake of the HIV-AIDS outbreak, advocates powerfully for interdisciplinary approaches to disease, emphasizing how outbreak narratives, both historically and in the twenty-first century, work to stigmatize nations, groups, and individuals. Yet as Ronald Schleifer and Jerry Vannatta remind us, the "chief concern of medicine" remains the co-creation of narratives about illness, pain, and suffering by patients

[5] See, for example, Bravermen, ed. (2023, 27–40); Slovic and Rangarajan, eds. (2022).

and their physicians; medical practice centers on talking to patients, trying to comprehend the specific etiologies of disease that evolve in these narratives (Schleifer and Vannatta 2013, 2019). Veterinarians, though, face the problem that their patients don't talk. Narratives of animal disease and suffering are always cast in the vocabularies of their owners, rescuers, shepherds, or herders. Even in the twenty-first century, with the "non-human turn," most scholars, Abigail Woods argues, "have not significantly revised their perception of what constitutes medical history" (14). This is a less a critique of the medical humanities, which will doubtless remain focused on human-centered experiences, than a reminder that we—doctors and patients and caretakers—share this planet with other animals. We marginalize or ignore animal plagues and nonhuman vectors at our own peril.

I use the term "medical posthumanities," then, as a way of nudging humanists toward a different starting point, the recognition that our biosphere includes not only humans and other mammals but birds, reptiles, trees, plants, and countless microbes. My version of the medical posthumanities, in this respect, is indebted both to the One Health movement and to what Stacy Alaimo has termed the "trans-corporeality" of existence, which presupposes interdependence between human health and that of the natural world (Alaimo 2010). As I described it in 2021, the medical posthumanities is less a doctrine than an opportunity to move beyond our disciplinary homes into "new subjectivities and political relations; as a multidisciplinary arena that takes transcorporeality rather than the animal, the human, or the machine as its ontological grounding and epistemological warrant, the medical posthumanities exists in the in-between" (Cole 2021b, 466). Since then, the term "medical posthumanities" has been circulating across several disciplines; a recent special issue on the medical posthumanities describes my initial framing as a "helpful starting point" for "examining posthuman health" in even "broader ways" (Crocker et al. 2023, 7). In whatever iteration—and I hope there are several—the remit of the medical posthumanities is to keep alive *relations* between and among seemingly different entities, practices, and phenomena, relations all too often occluded.

Let me offer a brief contemporary example of such occlusion. Writing in March 2020, at the beginning of the COVID-19 breakout, Stephen Greenblatt found in Lucretius's "Of the Nature of Things" a "radical materialism" that might serve as a model of the philosophical mindset during the imposed quarantines of coronavirus protocols. When things are not going well, he claims, when "the mutations of seed plagues bring disease and death," if one can still "keep calm, remain rational, and somehow find it possible to take pleasure in life" (2020) then one may have learned the lesson of Epicureanism. If Greenblatt, like Lucretius, is describing a philosophy, he is also describing an ecological and epidemiological event affecting species other than humans. In *De Rerum Natura*, Lucretius writes of "bane upgathering" that "kindles a devastation" on "races of men and herds of cattle." This pestilence falls upon the waters,

> Or settles on the very crops of grain
> Or other meat of men and feed of flocks.
> Or it remains a subtle force, suspense
> In the atmosphere itself; and when there from
> We draw our inhalations of mixed air,
> Into our body equally its bane
> Also we must suck in. In manner like,
> Oft comes the pestilence upon the kine,
> And sickness, too, upon the sluggish sheep. (2008, 6)

In Lucretius's account, because humans and other animals are vulnerable to corrupted air, water, grain, and meat, they are equally exposed to a "subtle force" that disrupts agricultural production, food supplies, human and, significantly, animal health. Greenblatt's Epicureanism, it is worth noting, sacrifices the multispecies nature of Lucretius's plague narrative to the demands of philosophical repose—or perhaps to the cosmopolitan demands of the *New Yorker*—in ways both inimical to ecological thought and, ironically, to what Lucretius has to say about a "pestilence" that falls on "kine," "sluggish sheep," and humans alike.

The medical posthumanities, by contrast, advocates for a multispecies awareness, and compels us to confront "the human" as a species that engineers—and often wreaks havoc—on a planetary scale. For scholars in the humanities, as Rosie Braidotti argues, this critique of anthropocentrism is highly demanding because it requires that we undertake a double shift, to understand ourselves *as* members of a species, and then the human *as one among many other* species (Braidotti 2013, 7–17). Moreover, to make this shift can be controversial and wrenching in part because for the formerly enslaved, for colonized peoples, for women, and for anyone disempowered ethnically and economically from power-sharing, the call for posthumanism may seem, at best, premature. "The human," after all, as Zakiyya Iman Jackson has reminded us, functions as a category of privilege (Jackson

2020, 3–14). Posthumanism has been accused with some justification of presentism (bad history), of flattening out distinctions among humans, animals, and things (bad humanities), and of papering over differences between the ecological impacts—indeed, the very humanity—of colonial powers and the peoples they subjugate. Having said that, posthumanism *can* attend to the more-than-human without blinding us to the stark realities of power differentials or how entire groups of people, again and again, have been consigned to the subhuman. Braidotti readily admits, and I agree, that posthumanism is an imperfect concept, but one that enables a wide range of research, attention to the more-than-human world, new and relational ways of thinking about cultural, ecological, and biophysical transformations. At best, an historically informed posthumanism enables us to talk across disciplines in ways that can lead to the articulation of new and more ecologically robust ethical values and political commitments.

The medical posthumanities, then, is a call for species-level thinking, a strategy we need to deal with the emergence of the complex medical, economic, and sociopolitical challenges of zoonotic disease: the COVID-19 pandemic, the Mpox virus, new strains of bird flu, and so on. Highly pathogenic versions of the latter have been enabled by the sheer number of vulnerable cattle on this planet. In a mere half-century, from 1961 to 2010, the global population of cattle slaughtered for food leapt from roughly 8 to 64 billion; by 2050, it is expected to double again (Patel and Moore 2018, 155). In India, where there are over 500 million livestock, the widespread use of diclofenac, used to treat pain and inflammation in cattle, resulted in a mass mortality of scavenging vultures, which itself led to a human public health emergency, an additional 100,000 deaths in regions with crashing vulture populations (Frank and Sudarshan 2024, 3007–3040). Even as zoonotic diseases reach a tipping point, as global food systems become increasingly fragile, the Trump administration in the United States has been actively destroying networks of scientific knowledge on which disease mitigation and food security depend.[6] Trying to

[6] Examples of Trump's destructive acts so far include withdrawing the United States from the World Health Organization, restricting research at the Centers for Disease Control, cutting funding at the National Institute of Health, decimating NOAA (National Oceanic and Atmospheric Administration), and installing disinformationist and vaccine sceptic Robert F. Kennedy Jr. as Secretary of Health and Human Services. See Stephanie Armour & KFF Health News, "Trump's Administration Will Attack Health Care from Multiple Angles," *Scientific American* November 7, 2024.

address this pestilential environment will require more than philosophy and more than attention to the human world. It will require us all—humanists, healers, farmers, and scientists—working together to preserve and share fundamental facts about science, disease, animal and environmental health. My contribution here is fairly specific: to offer a transdisciplinary history of cattle plagues and their real or imagined cross-contagions, thereby illuminating the shared vulnerability of humans and livestock in global cattle-grain regimes.

"Nor 'Scape the Beasts"

If art and literature can, as Greenblatt suggests, help us "keep calm," help us find "pleasure" amid a devastating pandemic, they can also help trace how we got here. On the one hand, cross-species plagues are staples of European historical and literary records, classical, Mosaic, and Christian.[7] Writing in the midst of three eighteenth-century outbreaks, Robert Dossie identifies murrains among the ancients in Aristotle, Cato, Plutarch, Virgil, Livy, and Columella; in Publius Flavius Vegetius (fourth century) and Charlemagne's secretary Eginardus (whose *Memoirs of Europe* were later satirized by Delariviere Manley); and, among early moderns, in Conrad Gesner, Ulisse Aldrovandi, the physician Girolamo Fracastoro, and the naturalist Ubbo Emmius (Dossie 1768, 372). Sudden and massive deaths of livestock, then, were central to how early modern Europeans understood both the ancient world and their own agricultural, theological, and economic systems. As I argue in subsequent chapters, Virgil's *Georgics* became a touchstone in the seventeenth and eighteenth centuries for discussions of animal disease, but his *Aeneid* includes an extremely influential description of the plague in Crete, a description recycled throughout the early modern period in literature and art. In book three of the *Aeneid*, on the advice of Anchises, Aeneus and the Trojans sail to Crete to build the city of Pergamea. Almost immediately, however, plague breaks out; the gods of Troy reveal to Aeneus that Anchises was mistaken about the

[7] Historical references to the bubonic plague are found in the *Iliad* of Homer (ca. 1000 BCE), as well as in the *History of the Peloponnesian War* of Thucydides (430–426 BCE), in the Bible's Book of Exodus, and in the *Metamorphoses* of Ovid (8 CE); references to anthrax are also found in the *Georgics* of Virgil (29 BCE), in *De Medicina* of Celsus (ca. 47 CE), in the *Naturalis Historia* of Pliny the Elder (77 CE) and in *De Differentiis Febrium* of Galen (ca. 200 CE). See Tanga et al. (2022: 213–49), and the articles by Dirckx (1981: 191–196); (2000a: 197–202); and (2000b: 459–464).

location of the city of "ancestors," which should have been erected in Italy, not Crete. The plague, then, is a measure of the gods' anger. This passage is the basis for Marcantonio Raimondi's copper engraving *Il Morbetto* (c. 1512), a work executed during a period marked by rinderpest and anthrax outbreaks in Italy.

Based on a design by Marcantonio's associate, Raphael, this engraving (Fig. 1.1) includes, in the background, a blasted field, a partially destroyed building, and a dead horse; in the foreground, juxtaposed, are two scenes of death and dying, one featuring humans and the other, hoofed animals. On the right, a child reaches for the breast of his dead mother, whose sight and smell disgust the people passing by her; on the left, a downed bull lies behind and slightly above a pile of fallen sheep in the foreground.

A pedestal with a quotation from *Aeneid* 3.140–41 splits the scene. Its various translations over the centuries help to illustrate how easy it is to

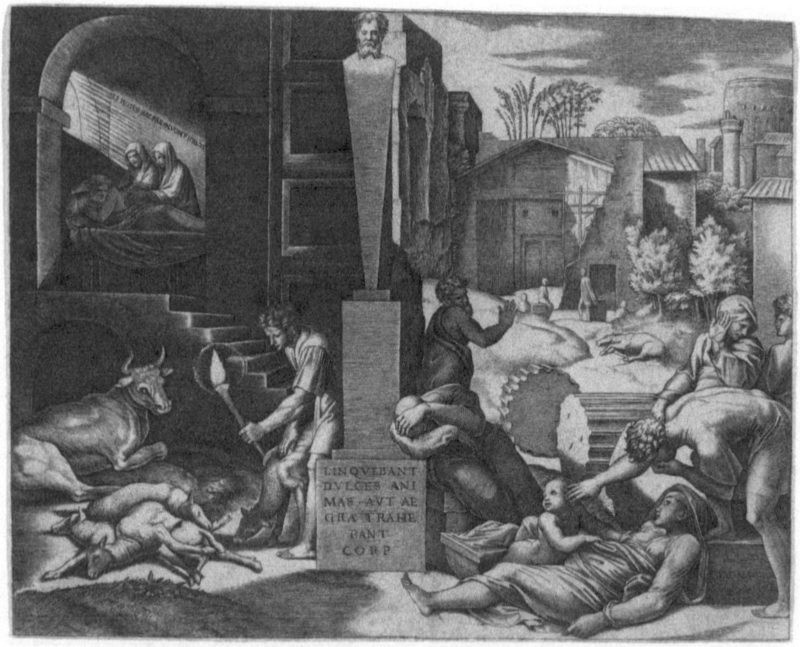

Fig. 1.1 Marcantonio Raimondi, *Il Morbetto (The Plague)*, c. 1512–/13. Courtesy of National Gallery of Art, Washington

erase the multispecies nature of plagues. H. Rushton Fairclough's early twentieth-century prose translation of this section renders "they"—the victims of the plague—as decidedly human: "of a sudden, from tainted quarter of the sky, came a pestilence and season of death, to the wasting of our bodies and the piteous ruin of trees and crops" (Virgil 1999, Bk. 3: 140–141). "Men gave up their sweet lives," the translation continues, "or dragged enfeebled frames; Sirius, too, scorched the fields with drought; the grass withered, and the sickly crop denied sustenance" (3: 141–142). No beasts are mentioned in Fairclough's translation at all. Instead, the plague is cast as a human crisis—a "season of death" apparently caused by or contemporaneous with a crop-killing drought. Yet the further we go back in time—the closer we get to the world of Marcantonio—the less anthropocentric translations of Virgil seem to be.[8] In Richard Stanyhurst's 1582 version of *The Aeneid*, a plague ranged "with foule contagion ayrye/ Both bodyes festring and fruict trees plentiful harming" (49). Here "both" links "bodyes" to "fruict trees" and leaves open the species identity of any sentient beings who are suffering. John Dryden's 1697 translation of the *Aeneid* takes advantage of this ambiguity in the Latin to depict a multispecies plague in keeping with Marcantonio's engraving. Dryden emphasizes "pestilential heat" as a cause of disease and invokes miasma theory: "When rising vapors choke the wholesome air," he writes,

> And blasts of noisome winds corrupt the year;
> The trees devouring caterpillars burn;
> Parch'd was the grass, and blighted was the corn;
> Nor 'scape the beasts; for Sirius, from on high,
> With pestilential heat infects the sky;
> My men—some fall, the rest in fevers fry. (Dryden 1987, 3: 191–196)

By specifying the afflicted bodies—"beasts" as well as Aeneas's "men"—Dryden casts in poetic form the interspecies contagion foregrounded by Marcantonio. Here Trojans are not the sole victims of "noisome winds" and "pestilential heat" but are part of a biosphere—domesticated livestock, trees, grass, corn—threatened by a catastrophe that includes, but extends beyond, contagious "fevers" to "fry" the human and more-than-human environment.

[8] Fairclough's contemporary, E. Fairfax Taylor (1907), uses the term "mortal limbs" rather than "our bodies": "Sweet life from mortals fled; they dropped and died" (65). Taylor's version is more in keeping with earlier English translations of Virgil.

Dryden's rendering, "Nor 'scape the beasts," reminds us that, in marginalizing or glossing over representations of multispecies plagues, we may be misreading our own histories—literary, cultural, and medical. By focusing only on human disease, suffering, and death, we too easily shunt aside what seemed obvious—often horrifyingly obvious—to writers and readers three or four centuries ago. To offer one example, James Tyrell's *General History of England* (1696), Volume One, includes in the subject index for "Plague" multispecies afflictions. (I have added the year of the outbreak, in brackets.)

> *Plague;* a very sore one in *Britain, when*, l. 3. p. 117. [664]
> *A great one over all the Isle of* Britain, *and then it went into* Ireland, l. 4. p. 190. [665]
> *A great Mortality both of Men and Beasts*, l. 5. p. 269. [869]
> *Another great one upon Men, and Murrain of Cattle*, Id. p. 302. [897]
> *A great Mortality of Men, and a very malignant Feaver in* London, l. 6. p. 4. [990]
> *A great Mortality of Cattle in* England, Id. p. 21. [986]
> *A great number of Cattle died; and by the Intemperance of the Season, the Fruits of the Earth were destroyed*, Id. p. 70. [1090]
> *So great a Murrain of all sorts of Cattle in* England, *that none could ever remember the like*, Id. p. 85 [1014] (Tyrell 1696, lxxii)

Above, multispecies plagues extend from Roman Britain through the reigns of Ethelbert and Alfred, to Harold, the last Anglo-Saxon King. Significantly, the same locution—"a great Mortality"—applies to plague in both humans and cattle. Indeed, in Tyrell's Index, "Murrain" and "Plague" are cross listed, treated as equivalent terms (lxvi). This linking underscores early modern perceptions of contagious disease: "Murrain" is derived from old French "morine," whose first definition is plague or pestilence, and its second, a carcass or body of a dead animal. In fact, the word "murrain" originally applied to diseases afflicting *both* people and animals, but by the sixteenth century, this use was already becoming archaic, pushed aside by multiple and sometimes competing causal explanations.

Consider in this context George Thomson's analysis of the plague outbreak in London. *Loimotomia; or, The pest anatomized* (1666) claims that when "unseasonable weather . . . infests us," "when multitude of Insects, as Toads, Froggs, Flies, Cimires, and divers poysonous Creatures appear; when Cattle perish in great Numbers by some Contagious lues; when malignant Diseases, as Small Pox, Spotted Feavers; Scurvy, or the like, are frequent among us," then human plague will follow (1666, 54). According to a 1721 etymological dictionary, the word "lues" refers primarily to pestilence or plague, and secondarily to murrain; for Thomson, then, human and cattle plague are both semantically and causally linked (Bailey 1721, s.v. "lues"). Yet this relationship exists as part of a more populous network of potential actors—weather, insects, vermin, other diseases, such as "Scurvy"—any combination of which might be involved in a mortal outbreak. It is easy to extract from Thomson's chain of observed and linked phenomena an incipient understanding of agrilogistics: climate disruptions generate a "multitude of Insects" and vermin ("poisonous Creatures") who carry infection and destroy crops; cattle in "great Numbers" succumb to disease and malnutrition; humans, weakened by disease outbreaks, fall victim to the plague. Although nothing in Thomson's catalogue functions as what we might now recognize as a specific disease vector—say, fleas or lice carrying plague between mammals—a pestilential environment precedes disease outbreaks in humans and cattle alike. Two hundred years later, after Britain's third great plague of rinderpest (1855–56), George Fleming, trying to encourage the development of comparative pathology, similarly describes the intersections of human and animal disease, this time in unequivocal terms: for the medical historian, "it has been a matter of common observation from the earliest times," he writes, "that widespread pestilence in plants, and murrain in animals, have frequently either preceded, accompanied, or followed closely on those visitations which caused mortality and mourning in the habitations of men" (Fleming 1871, xxxii). Infested plants and infected livestock are deeply entangled in human disease and suffering.

Such early causal explanations, I shall argue, are rarely unyoked from Christian disease ecologies, and especially from notions of divine displeasure. Thomas Brooks, a popular seventeenth-century Puritan divine who stayed in London during the plague of 1666 to look after his flocks, claims that some physicians "ascribe [plague] to the heat of the Air," and some to "driness"; sometimes they blame it on "corruption" of the air and sometimes on "mens blood"; sometimes "Satan, and sometimes to the malignancy of the Planets" (Brooks 1666, 4–5). He insists, however, physicians are "of no value" unless they look beyond these "second causes, to the First Cause," to "*the wheel within the wheel*":

> The Plague is a hidden thing, a secret thing; it is a sickness, a disease, that more immediately comes from God, than any other sickness or disease doth.

> *Behold the hand of the Lord is upon thy cattel which is in the field, upon the horses, upon the asses, upon the camels, upon the oxen, and upon the sheep, there shall be a very grievous murrain.* (7)

For Brooks and many of his contemporaries, etiological differences between human and animal plague, murrains and pestilence, collapse under the rubric of "First Causes," or divine retribution. Brooks explicitly identifies human and animal disease as two aspects of the same punishment: "The word here [in Exodus 9:3] translated *murrain*, is in *chap.* 5. *v.* 3. termed *pestilence;* and it is one and the same disease, though when it is applied to cattel, it be usually rendred by murrain, yet when 'tis applied to men, as in the Scripture last cited, it is commonly called the pestilence" (6). By sweeping (human) pestilence and (animal) murrain—a pandemic and an epizootic—under the general category of "plague," Brooks subsumes differences between the human and more-than-human, even as he holds a sinful humanity responsible for bringing about both murrains and pestilence: "it [plague] more immediately comes from God, than any other sickness or disease doth." In such accounts, Christianity and medical discourse are caught up in scourge logic—the metanarrative of divine punishment for sin—and consequently in outbreak narratives: domesticated animals are, at once, the suffering victims of sinful sovereigns and nations and themselves agents in widespread ecological and socioeconomic disruption.

The Fifth Plague and Agrotheology

The biblical allusion in my title, *The Fifth Plague: Cattle, Contagion, and the Medical Posthumanities*, though, is intended to call attention to the outsized influence that the Exodus narrative played in structuring understandings of mass mortality events well into the Victorian era. At least between 1500 and 1900—and maybe even now—agriculture in Europe remained deeply entangled with Judeo-Christian theology, most obviously through the ten plagues of Egypt: the Nile being turned to blood, swarms of frogs, lice, flies, and locusts, boils, hail and fire, darkness, and the death of first-born sons (Cole 2016, 49–79). In Exodus (9:1–7), the fifth plague is an affliction or pestilence of livestock: "If [the Pharoah] refuse[s] to let [the Jews] go and continue[s] to hold them back, the hand of the Lord will bring a terrible plague on your livestock in the field—on your horses and donkeys and camels and on your cattle and sheep and goats." When Pharoah refuses, "all the livestock of Egypt died, but of the livestock of the sons of Israel, not one died."[9] The Exodus narrative, then, emphasizes the differential effects of animal plagues, treating murrains as multispecies outbreaks, while defining the medico-cultural bounds of Mosaic history that resonate throughout the early modern era and beyond. Plagues, including animal plagues, are evidence of God's anger or a divine desire to scourge a recalcitrant or fallen people, bringing them to heel.

As a visual representation of early modern agrotheology, consider an illustration from the 1572 edition of the Wittenberg Bible, which sold about 100,000 copies in the first 40 years after its initial 1534 printing. The woodcut (Fig. 1.2) combines the fifth and sixth plagues (the plague of boils). Animals of different kinds—horses, asses, oxen, sheep—are

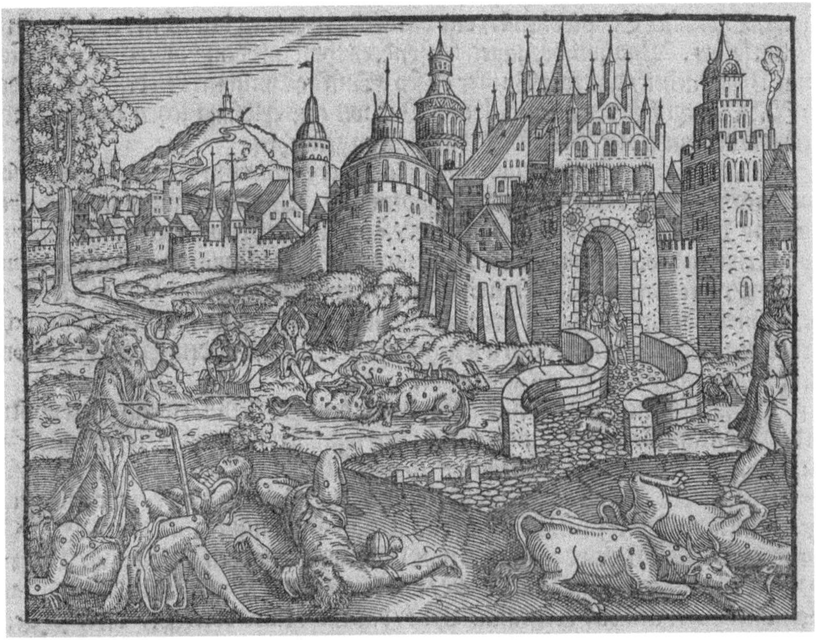

Fig. 1.2 *VI Plage. Bible, das ist. Die gantze heilige Schrifft.* Illustrator Johann Teufel. Courtesy of the Houghton Library, Harvard

[9]English translations of the Bible typically use the word *murrain* to describe the fifth plague, a term widespread in the ancient and medieval world (Sanskrit *mr*, Latin *mori*), and its equivalent also appears in many romance languages (Italian *moria*, French *murie*). See Fleming (1871, xxvii).

down. Even dogs lie dead on the cobblestone walk. People exist in various stages of affliction, some writhing on the ground, some still ambulatory. One common feature dominates this illustration, though: both human and animal bodies are covered by pustules or buboes of the same size. In ways that complicate the usual order of affliction—murrain precedes human mortalities—Teufel's art implies that the cattle and the people suffer the same infection. To the right and behind this epidemiological tragedy stand several well-dressed humans in the archway of the castle, observing or likely quarantining themselves from the peasants whose proximity to the dying animals marks them as part of a rural economy. Visually, the ruined agricultural economy represented by the dead cattle portends the death or financial ruin of the humans whose livelihoods depend on them. As one clergyman put it in a 1669 sermon, the fifth plague must be seen as a shared affliction: "It is hard to say, whether the dying groans of Beasts and Horses, or the Cryes of the Husband-men, and Carriers, or those whose livlyhoods was swept away by this Beasom [broom] of destruction was the greater" (Harrington 1669, 402).

In their sensitivity to the cascading effects of cross-species contagion and suffering, early modern artists and writers demonstrate a kind of incipient, if theologized, awareness of the more-than-human world that One Health and ecological scholars, in very different ways, are working to recapture and update. Biblical scholars and scientists, past and present, have had a field day trying to pinpoint a specific disease characterized by skin eruptions that could strike both men and livestock; candidates include anthrax, leprosy, smallpox, a staph infection, boils from a stable fly, and cancer caused by soot.[10] The microbiologist Siro Trevisanato claims that toxic ash, loaded with cinnabar, could have poisoned the ancient Nile. Frogs then would have left in search of clean water, leaving insects to lay eggs in the bodies of the human and nonhuman dead; these larvae and then adult insects could have been possible sources of infection (Trevisanto 2005). As late as 1996, the epidemiologist John S. Marr argues that red algae killed fish and turned the Nile's water crimson, prompting frogs to go in search of food, which meant they were not eating insects, so that flies, lice, and locusts proliferated. He suggests that the lice (third plague)

[10] See, for example, C. J. Humphreys (2003, 125–28); Cassuto (2005, 113–14); and Mazokopakis and Karagiannis (2019: 310–13).

and flies (fourth plague) may have included *culicoides*, which can cause African horse sickness and Bluetongue—the Fifth Plague—but also the outbreak of boils, which is a common symptom of glanders (Marr and Malloy 1996, 7–24). The temptation to engage in such retrospective diagnosis—to which many veterinary historians occasionally succumb—is ever present.

That said, I am less interested in diagnosing specific diseases than I am in understanding how early Christian disease ecologies helped shape human-animal relationships in cattle-grain economies. In this sense, *The Fifth Plague* extends the project I began in *Imperfect Creatures: Vermin, Literature, and the Sciences of Life, 1600–1740*: to examine how "vermin," broadly conceived, helped structure ways of thinking about the health of a body politic vulnerable to hunger, disease, and famine, thereby helping to define what it meant to be human. If vermin are, as I have argued, the constitutive *outside* of Judeo-Christian agrotheology—no vermin, after all, were allowed on Noah's ark—cattle are its constitutive center, the spine of its theological, economic, and sociopolitical imperatives. The status of cattle as animal laborer, food source, and living commodity (as in the wool industry) made murrains a matter of grave national economic concern; beef eating by the eighteenth century, for example, had become such a well-known marker of Englishness that threats to cattle and meat consumption were perceived by many as threats to national identity (Rogers 2003). During the first year of a rinderpest or anthrax outbreak, some 70% of cattle can die, often tens or even hundreds of thousands, leading to food shortages and massive economic dislocations (Cole 2021a, 35–53). Always threats to grain economies, vermin, broadly conceived, also played mysterious roles in murrains. In the period covered by *The Fifth Plague*, the agents and the means of contagion were, as we saw in the *Aeneid* and Exodus, speculative and multiple: they included air, to be sure, but also insects, water, heat, grass, toads, or—more generally—putrefaction, the effluvia from bodies that have fallen victim to disease. *Imperfect Creatures* and *The Fifth Plague* function as complementary analyses of cattle-grain economies in relation to Biblical disease ecologies.

Caught in what Morton calls the epidemic "feedback loop" of agrilogistics, transported across greater and greater distances to satisfy an ever-growing European demand for meat, cattle and oxen in the early modern era were both carriers of contagious diseases and their most frequent casualties (Morton 2016; Morton 2017, 91–111), Cattle; in other words, occupy double roles as enzootic vector, infecting the herd, and as enzootic victim.

Even more frightening for humans, the jury was decidedly out on whether cattle could serve as sources of disease capable of crossing species bounds. Many writers—deeply influenced by the Exodus accounts—contended with both the terrifying *scale* of cattle disease and its real or imaginary *proximity* to human diseases. As the intimacy between dead livestock and dying people in Teufel's Wittenberg Bible engraving demonstrates, cattle plagues were yoked to bubonic plague because both killed on massive scales and in devastating numbers. Later, during the eighteenth century, cattle outbreaks would be compared to smallpox, and by the nineteenth-century, increasingly to cholera. Thus debates about the uncertain lines dividing humans from animals between 1500 and 1900 are not only about human exceptionalism. Instead—or in addition to—they register the confusion, alarm, displacements, and adaptations caused by mass mortality events as they played out in a world increasingly shaped by the climate instability of the Little Ice Age, global trade, and imperial expansion. Read in this context, the ten plagues of Egypt helped promote the not-unfounded fear that cattle afflictions could be conveyed directly to human populations; equally important, they helped establish the source of disease as "elsewhere"—Africa, to be sure, but also Hungary, Eurasia, and later the Russian steppes. Through murrain discourse, alien ecologies became identified as geopolitical sources of contagion, their people and animals designated as what Christos Lynteris terms "epidemic villains" subject to plague containment or even eradication policies (Lynteris 2019, 5–9).

We now have a word for cross-species transmission—zoonosis—as well as the ability to distinguish between, say, bacteria and viruses, essential knowledge for tracing disease vectors. Because I sometimes use contemporary language to describe disease phenomena expressed in radically different ways before 1900, it may be helpful to distinguish among a few key terms here. General speaking, "zoonotic" or "enzootic" refers to transfer of disease *between beings*, and "epizootic" to *how many beings* are afflicted. Although the term "zoonotic disease" was not coined until the nineteenth century, the recognition that nonhumans could carry diseases and transmit them to humans, as we have seen, goes back for centuries, if not millennia. Technically, zoonotic diseases are transmittable across species, even when that transfer involves a non-vertebrate disease vector. Such diseases can be conveyed by inhalation (anthrax); ingestion (salmonella, brucellosis); animal bites (rabies); exposure of skin (leptospirosis, fleas); and through arthropods (Lyme disease). Although diseases like rabies, malaria, HIV-AIDS, and now COVID have garnered the most headlines, a host of diseases can be transferred between cattle and humans, primarily by ingesting tainted milk or meat: these include anthrax, brucellosis, leptospirosis, rabies, ringworm, salmonellosis, and tuberculosis. Even syphilis is regarded as zoonotic, spreading from cattle and sheep to humans, originally perhaps by sexual transmission (Lynteris, 58).

The terms "epizootic" and "panzootic," in contrast, refer not to modes of transmission but matters of scale. The former ("epizootic") corresponds to "epidemic" in human medicine, and the latter ("panzootic") to "pandemic." African swine fever, at the moment, is classified as a panzootic, having spread from Africa in 2005, to Eastern Europe (2007), to the EU (2014), to parts of Asia (2018), and to Oceania (2020); after an absence of nearly forty years, it shortly thereafter reappeared first in North America and then on the Italian mainland.[11] African swine fever is not, however, regarded as zoonotic, although humans may serve as a disease vector, carrying it on their clothes. Rinderpest—the most immediately fatal form of cattle plague—can be characterized as epizootic or panzootic (and sometimes both) depending on the perception of its range and mortality. It is generally agreed that the Mongol invasion of Europe in the thirteenth century initiated a panzootic in Europe, and another occurred in 1709 by virtue of Venetian trade with the east. In the 1880s, rinderpest was introduced to Africa by cattle imported from India to feed Italian troops; sweeping through the continent, this panzootic "wiped out 90% of the domestic cattle and wild buffalo" (Barrett 2008, 504). Although rinderpest can be spread through contaminated clothing, feed, and equipment, and is caused by a morbillivirus closely related to human measles, it cannot be spread to humans.[12] Rinderpest is nevertheless zoonotic, strictly speaking, in that it can be spread between different species of animals, wild or domestic, through aerosolized droplets and bodily secretions. Anthrax can affect humans as well as grazing animals, such as sheep, but tends not to be responsible for mass mortality events—in other words, tends *not* to be epizootic—especially across large geographical areas. Before germ theory, epizootics and panzootics like rinderpest were never fully distinguished

[11] https://www.woah.org/en/disease/african-swine-fever/#ui-id-2, accessed December 28, 2023.

[12] It is possible that a type of rinderpest once existed in the human population but then became measles in the Early Middle Ages; its predecessor, an "ancestral morbillivirus," possibly jumped back and forth between human and bovine populations, killing both, before burning itself out. See Newfield (2015: 1–38). For a longer, foundational account of premodern cattle plague, see Newfield (2024, 235–284).

from pandemics like the bubonic plague; both can become enzootic (in the case of rinderpest), or endemic (in the case of bubonic plague), even though all were cast, as Brooks notes, under the rubric "pestilence" or, when referring specifically to animals, "murrain."

Reading Zoonotically

Although mass bovine graves indicate at least two major plague events occurred during the medieval period—one in the sixth century and one in the tenth—the following chapters follow the chronology of European and especially British cattle plague outbreaks. Sporadic outbreaks in the fifteenth, sixteenth, and seventeenth centuries (Chaps. 2 and 3) gave way, in the eighteenth century, to several distinct epizootics in France and England (Chaps. 4 and 5); its spread accelerated by steam ships and railway systems, cattle plague returned to Great Britain in 1865 and 1866 (Chap. 6) before breaking out in India. I focus on western Europe in this study not because animal plagues are exclusive to the region but because imperialism created demands for meat and forms of transportation that accelerated the circulation of cattle disease, ensuring that it became—and still remains—a global phenomenon. *The Fifth Plague* is structured more or less chronologically, but that order should not set up expectations for a straightforward veterinary history. In researching and writing this study, I have tried hard not to repeat—at least not at great length—accounts that can be found elsewhere. Instead, I have been drawn to problems that are important to animal studies, ecology, literature, and a medical posthumanities. Chief among these is how animal disease (zoonotic or not) shapes relations. The category of "relations" is intended to be expansive. It includes without being limited to Christian ethnocentrism, anthropocentrism, and pastoral biopolitics; meat markets and nationalism; eco-anxiety, necropolitics, and plague policy, which involves the capture of cattle within an international eco-medical regime.

Ultimately, *The Fifth Plague* is about shared afflictions. Leonard Mascall, author of *The first booke of cattell*, which appeared in 1596, describes cattle plague as "a marvelous infection," a term that adequately captures the destructive, confusing, reason-defying outbreaks of the sixteenth and seventeenth centuries. Chapter 2 focuses, in part, on a 1612 Latin edition of a fourth-century poem on cattle plague, *Carmen Bucolicum De Mortibus*

Boum [The Bucolic Song On the Deaths of Cattle].[13] I have included the first English translation of these verses in the Appendix. Dialogue among the poem's three speakers—Aegon, Buculus, and Tityrus—offers a poignant description of the material and psychological consequences of cattle plague. The poem ends with a Christianized deus ex machina: after Tityrus brands crosses on the foreheads of his cattle, his herd miraculously escapes the plague that plunged both Aegon and Buculus into despair and financial ruin. *De Mortibus Boum* introduces concerns that recur throughout subsequent chapters: the limits of animal husbandry in treating murrain; the economic devastation of farmers whose livestock sicken and die; the "bovine elegy" as a rural lament for stricken animals; the role of Christian apologetics; and the ways in which multiple disease vectors and causal mechanisms get swept under the rubric of miasma theory. Among these multiple disease vectors are insects, and the second part of this chapter explores real and perceived relationships between entomology and epidemiology in the early modern era. Insects exist (alongside earthquakes, cold blasts, and infected air) in classical and Biblical literature as a popular causal agent of plague; in Exodus, as we have seen, they are straightforward disease vectors. Equally important, though, in an age before a scientific understanding of microbial disease vectors emerged, swarming insects or traveling infestations provided a means to visualize—and theorize—how contagious diseases could spread from region to region and even country to country. In this context, I reexamine connections between *De Mortibus Boum* and John Pory's English translation of Leo Africanus's *A geographical history of Africa* (1600), which includes *History Against the Pagans* and historical accounts of locust infestation. Pory's translation shares with *De Mortibus Boum* a tendency to divide the world into "Christian" and "Pagan," the latter represented by swarming insects, divine scourges for sinful peoples and nations.

Chapter 3, "Zoonotic Shakespeare: Merchants and Livestock in Venice," rereads a canonical literary text from the perspective of the medical posthumanities. In ways seldom discussed, Shakespeare's *The Merchant of Venice* provides telling evidence of the global trade in livestock—Venice was the center of the eastern Mediterranean cattle trade—and correspondent networks of contagion. Building on the work of Bruce Boehrer, Laurie Shannon, Andrew McRae, and other scholars working in the early

[13]The text is described by Phillips in *Theatarum Poetarum* (1675): "*Endeleichus,* otherwise called *Severus Sanctus,* a Rhetorician of an uncertain time, whose Eclogue about the death of *Oxen,* is extant in the Collection set forth by *Pithaeus*" (73).

modern period, I reconsider some key passages in the play, many about sheep, in the context of the disease outbreaks that devastated both Italy and England. These outbreaks set in motion a set of rigorous protocols adopted by the Venetian Senate for isolating infected animals, quarantining herds, halting cattle shipments, and, in some cases, prophylactically slaughtering herds in danger of being infected. To read Shakespeare—who was, after all, the son of a leather tanner—in light of his knowledge of cattle and the cattle trade is to confront, in unexpected ways, perspectives on the real and imagined cross-species infections often glossed over by anthropocentric literary interpretations. I call this historical, transdisciplinary practice "reading zoonotically." Central to this chapter and to the play as a whole are tensions between Christian pastoral power and growing fears about an amoral, or even immoral, animal trade driven by greed, violence, and exclusion.

Between 1711 and 1769, more than 200 million cattle in Western Europe succumbed to a variety of diseases (Spinage 2003, 5). A growing international cattle trade ensured that pandemics became transnational epidemiological and ecological crises. According to Cindy Ermus, epidemics "were now described not only in terms of divine vengeance or celestial movements or prodigies, but increasingly as products of commercial activity" (Ermus 2023, 5). This is clearly the case in Daniel Defoe's writings, which are characterized by a split between his knowledge of the cattle trade, along with the infections it could entail, and his desire to project any such disease onto an alien and "pagan" other—notably the "Tartars." In Chap. 4, "Journals of the Plague Years: Flesh Markets and Easterly Winds," I begin by examining depictions of cattle plague in treatises about the 1720 bubonic plague at Marseilles which, significantly, was preceded by scattered outbreaks of cattle disease. These treatises include Richard Bradley's *The Plague at Marseilles Consider'd, with Remarks Upon the Plague in General, Shewing Its Cause and the Nature of Infection* (1721) and Nathaniel Hodges's updated *Loimologia, or An Historical Account of the Plague that Raged in London, 1665* (1720). While such works consider at length purported relationships between murrains and bubonic plague, Defoe's texts downplay the possibility of multispecies contagion, except by unsuspecting people eating contaminated meat. A deep anxiety about meat and meat markets runs through Defoe's *Due Preparations for the Plague* (1722) and *Journal of the Plague Year* (1722), especially meat imported from the Eurasian steppes. These eastern lands, with their huge herds of horses, sheep, cattle, and camels, began, in the seventeenth century, to occupy the geo-pathological position earlier represented by a presumably noxious Nile Delta. I examine reports of what was probably anthrax in travel writers in the seventeenth and eighteenth centuries, linking those to Defoe's derogatory comments about "Tartars" in his plague writings, and to Crusoe's dramatic attack on the Tartar "idol" Cham Chi-Thaungu, in *Farther Adventures of Robinson Crusoe* (1719). If his novels and nonfiction prose exhibit a detailed knowledge of the international cattle trade, Defoe nonetheless believes that physical corruption is a sign of moral corruption, and he projects fears of contagion from the east onto what he imagines as a "filthy" alien other.

The fifth chapter, "1740–1790: Bovine Elegies and Bioinsecurities," returns to the issue of ecological vulnerability raised in *De Mortibus Boum*. By the mid-eighteenth century, cattle plague had become endemic in the Netherlands, and threatened to do the same in England. Robert Dossie's influential *Memoirs of Agriculture and other Oeconomical Arts* published in 1768 (with volume two following three years later), during England's third eighteenth-century outbreak, treats cattle plague as a "very momentous national evil" against which the government must provide "a means of security" (Dossie 1771, 367). His views were shared widely during these decades. I analyze hymns, sermons, topical poetry, newspapers, and natural histories, and eighteenth-century versions of the "bovine elegy" to examine these epidemiological threats and the challenges they posed for contemporary writers, farmers, physicians, and government officials. Dossie was one of many agriculture writers who, partly out of desperation, partly driven by a desire to cut economic losses, began to question the efficacy of cull and bury policies, a long-standing tool of government plague containment and control. He argues that cattle plague is seasonal and therefore partly subject to the ministrations of good husbandry. While his turn away from cull to cure might be perceived as a sign of increased concern about animal welfare, I treat it as the paradoxical capture of cattle within an instrumental medico-economic regime. Separated from "Nature" in the public imagination, while still serving as disease vectors and victims, dying cattle provoked complex responses, from disinterest to affective, elegiac compassion. The chapter ends by considering the possibility that eighteenth-century eco-anxiety includes not only climate-related disaster but the trauma of mass animal die offs.

My final chapter focuses mostly on the years 1865 and 1866, when, after a series of epizootic events on the continent, cattle plague returned to England. In contrast to eighteenth-century writers, as Lyon Playfair's

1866 *The Cattle Plague in Its Relation to Past Epidemics and to the Present Attack* attests, many nineteenth-century physicians and politicians brought to cattle plague knowledge about infection and sanitary practices gained through a century of fighting cholera outbreaks in human populations. Although "Steppe Disease and Cholera During Britain's Last Great Outbreak" reprises many of the discourses featured in previous chapters (insects as disease vectors, the bovine elegy, and pastoral politics), I focus here on the constitutive functions of a mistaken analogy between cholera and rinderpest. For many members of the public, the analogy helped provide support for disease mitigation measures they could set against traditional culling and killing policies. The effect of this analogy on the fate of potentially and actually infected cattle, however, was contradictory. On the one hand, drawing on lessons from cholera, the sanitary movement brought about better conditions (clean water, mucked stalls, roomier train cars) for cattle being raised or transported to market; on the other hand, cattle became more deeply embedded in the imperial logics of import theory and steppe disease: namely, the belief that "foreign" cattle or "alien" husbandry practices, rather than the local cattle market or a divinely sanctioned meat-based diet, were responsible for epizootics and panzootics. I explore arguments about cholera, rinderpest, and plague mitigation policy in popular magazines, including *Punch*, in well-known medical treatises, and through a satirical anti-contagionist text. This chapter ends with a brief analysis of what is, to my knowledge, the only English novel on cattle plague. *The Days of the Cattle Plague*, Sophie Amelia Prosser's 1872 novel, set in a dairy farming community south of Cheshire and published by the Religious Tract Society, updates Christian agrotheology for British readers in the nineteenth century.

In *Quick Cattle and Dying Wishes: People and their Animals in Early Modern England*, Erica Fudge argues that complex relationships between early modern humans and their livestock are lost in our collective tendency to reduce these animals "to little more than the machines of (human) history" (Fudge 2018, 15). Good husbandry, she demonstrates, "might best be found in actions that are difficult to trace as they have left little record because they were so ordinary" (64)—actions such as talking to, patting, worrying about the health and well-being of animals vital to rural and national economies. Nothing in my study undermines this important claim. But pastoral politics exercised in the midst of repeated epidemics and on an increasingly industrial scale necessarily involved government interventions, plague bureaucracies, and calculations about the value of bovine life and death through which potentially infected livestock became, sadly, things, earlier iterations of potentially infected meat.[14] *The Fifth Plague: Cattle, Contagion, and the Medical Posthumanities* tries to narrate how this fitful, partial, and ongoing transformation from animal to meat, living subject to living object, occurs, and why—especially now—it should matter to humanists.

References

Alaimo, Stacy. 2010. *Bodily Natures: Science, Environment, and the Material Self.* Bloomington: Indiana University Press.

American Veterinary Medical Association. 2008. *One Health: A New Professional Imperative*, 2. https://www.avma.org/sites/default/files/resources/one-health_final.pdf.

Armour, Stephanie, and KFF Health News. 2024. Trump's Administration Will Attack Health Care from Multiple Angles. *Scientific American*. November 7.

Bailey, Nathan. 1721. *An Universal Etymological English Dictionary*. London: Printed for E. Bell, J. Darby, et al.

Bar-On, Yinon M., Rob Phillips, and Ron Milo. 2018. The Biomass Distribution on Earth. *PNAS* 115 (25): 6506–6511.

Barrett, T. 2008. Rinderpest and Distemper Viruses. In *Encyclopedia of Virology*, ed. Brian W. J. Mahy and Marc H. V. Van Regenmortel, 3rd ed., 497–507. Amsterdam: Academic Press.

Braidotti, Rosi. 2013. *The Posthuman*. London: Polity.

Bravermen, Irus, ed. 2023. *More Than-One-Health: Humans, Animals, and Environment Post-Covid*. New York: Routledge.

Brooks, Thomas. 1666. *A heavenly cordial for all those servants of the Lord that have had the plague*. London: John Hancock.

Brown, Karen, and Daniel Gilfoyle, eds. 2010. *Healing the Herds: Disease, Livestock Economies, and the Globalization of Veterinary Medicine*. Athens, OH: Ohio University Press.

Cassidy, Angela. 2016. One Medicine? Advocating (Inter)disciplinarity at the Interfaces of Animal Health, Human Health, and the Environment. In *Investigating Interdisciplianry Collaboration: Theory and Practice Across Disciplines*, ed. S. Frickel, M. Albert, and B. Prainsack, 213–235. New Brunswick, NJ: Rutgers University Press.

[14] Exceptions do exist. See Govindrajan's excellent study (2018) based on field work in Uttarakhand, India.

Cassidy, Angela. 2019. *Vermin, Victims, and Disease: British Debates over Bovine Tuberculosis and Badgers*. London: Palgrave Macmillan.

Cassuto, U. 2005 (rpt). *A Commentary on the Book of Exodus*. Translated by Israel Abrahams. Jerusalem: Magnes Press of Hebrew University.

Chico, Tita. 2019. From Fleece to Fleets; or, Wool and the Production of Wonder. *Eighteenth-Century Fiction* 32:101–121.

Cole, Lucinda. 2016. *Imperfect Creatures: Vermin, Literature, and the Sciences of Life, 1600–1740*. Ann Arbor: University of Michigan Press.

Cole, Lucinda. 2021a. What Is an Animal? Contagion and Being Human in a Multispecies World. *Lumen* 40:35–53.

Cole, Lucinda. 2021b. Aliens, Plagues, One Health, and the Medical Posthumanities. *Configurations* 29 (4): 453–467.

Crocker, Rosalind, Mary Dawson, Eva Surawy, and Shauna Walker. 2023. Introduction: Medical Posthumanities: Reassessing and Reimagining the Human. *Interconnections: Journal of Posthumanism* 2 (2): 4–13.

Dirckx, J. H. 1981. Virgil on Anthrax. *American Journal of Dermatopathology* 3:191–196.

Dirckx, J. H. 2000a. Pestilence Narratives in Classical Literature: A Study in Creative Imitation: I. Homer, Sophocles, Thucydides, and Lucretius. *American Journal of Dermatopathology* 22:197–202.

Dirckx, J. H. 2000b. Pestilence Narratives in Classical Literature: A Study in Creative Imitation. II. Virgil, Ovid, Seneca, and Silius Italicus. *American Journal of Dermatopathology* 22:459–464.

Dossie, Robert. 1768. *Memoirs of Agriculture and other Oeconomical Arts*. London: J. Nourse.

Dossie, Robert. 1771. *Memoirs of Agriculture, and other Oeconomical Arts*. Vol. II. London: Printed for J. Nourse.

Dryden, John. 1987. In *The Works of John Dryden, Volume 5: Poems, The Works of Virgil in English 1697*, ed. William Frost. Berkeley: University of California Press.

Dyer, John. 2019. In *The Fleece*, ed. John Goodridge and Juan Christian Pellicer. Derby: USK Electronic Editions.

Ermus, Cindy. 2023. *The Great Plague Scare of 1720: Disaster and Diplomacy in the Eighteenth-Century Atlantic World*. Cambridge: Cambridge University Press.

Fleming, George. 1871. *Animal Plagues: Their History, Nature, and Prevention*. London: Chapman and Hall.

Frank, Eyal, and Anant Sudarshan. 2024. The Social Costs of Keystone Species Collapse: Evidence from The Decline of Vultures in India. *Amercian Economic Review* 114 (10): 3007–3040.

Fudge, Erica. 2018. *Quick Cattle and Dying Wishes: People and Their Animals in Early Modern England*. Ithaca: Cornell University Press.

Govindrajan, Radhika. 2018. *Animal Intimacies: Interspecies Relatedness in India's Central Himalayas*. Chicago: University of Chicago Press.

Greenblatt, Stephen. 2020. Invisible Bullets: What Lucretius Taught Us About Pandemics. *The New Yorker*. March 16.

Harrington, James. 1669. *A holy oyl; and, a sweet perfume taken out of the sanctuary of the most sacred scriptures*. London: Printed for the Author.

Humphreys, Colin J. 2003. *The Miracles of Exodus: A Scientist's Discovery of the Extraordinary Natural Causes of the Biblical Stories*. New York: Harper Collins.

Hüntelmann, Christian Jaser, Mieke Roscher, and Nadir Weber. 2024. Introduction: Animals and Epidemics in Historical Perspective. In *Animals and Epidemics: Interspecies Entanglements in Historical Perspective*, ed. Axel C. Huntelmann, Christian Mieke Jaser, Roscher, and Nadir Weber, 9–31. Köln: Böhlau.

Jackson, Zakiyyah Iman. 2020. *Becoming Human: Matter and Meaning in an Antiblack World*. New York: NYU Press.

King, Lonnie J., Larry R. Andersen, et al. 2008. Executive Summary of the AMVA One Health Initiative Task Force Report. *Journal of the American Veterinary Medical Association* 223 (2): 259–261.

Latour, Bruno. 1987. *Science in Action: How to Follow Scientists and Engineers through Society*. Cambridge: Harvard University Press.

Leonard, Mascall. 1587. *The first booke of cattell*. London: John Wolfe.

Lucretius. 2008. *De Rerum Natura: The Latin Text of Lucretius*. Edited and Translated by William Ellery Leonard and Stanley Barney Smith. Madison: University of Wisconsin Press.

Lynteris, Christos, ed. 2019. *Framing Animals as Epidemic Villains*. London: Palgrave Macmillan.

Marr, John S., and C. D. Malloy. 1996. An Epidemiologic Analysis of the Ten Plagues of Egypt. *Caduceus* 12:7–24.

Mazokopakis, E. E., and C. G. Karagiannis. 2019. Environmental and Medical Aspects Related to the Sixth Plague of Egypt. *Maedica* 14 (3): 310–313.

McDaniel, C. J., D. M. Cardwell, R. B. Moeller Jr., and C. G. Gray. 2014. Humans and Cattle: A Review of Bovine Zoonoses. *Vector Borne Zoonotic Diseases* 14 (1): 1–19.

McNeill, William H. 1977. *Plagues and Peoples*. New York: Random House.

McRae, Andrew. 1996. *God Speed the Plough: The Representation of Agrarian England, 1500–1660*. Cambridge: Cambridge University Press.

Menely, Tobias. 2021. *Climate and the Making of Worlds: Toward a Geohistorical Poetics*. Chicago: University of Chicago Press.

Milne, Anne. 2008. *Lactilla Tends Her Fav'rite Cow: Ecocritical Readings of Animals and Women in Eighteenth-Century British Labouring-Class Women's Poetry*. Lewisburg, PA: Bucknell University Press.

Morton, Timothy. 2016. *Dark Ecology: For a Logic of Future Coexistence*. New York: Columbia University Press.

Morton, Timothy. 2017. Why Ecological Awareness is Loopy. In *Imagining Earth: Concepts of Wholeness in Cultural Constructions of Our Home Planet*, ed. Solveig Nitzke and Nicolas Pethes, 91–111. Bielefeld: Transcript Verlag.

Newfield, Timothy P. 2015. Human–Bovine Plagues in the Early Middle Ages. *The Journal of Interdisciplinary History* 46 (1): 1–38.

Newfield, Timothy P. 2024. Premodern European Animal Plagues: Common but Enigmatic? In *Animals and Epidemics: Interspecies Entanglements in Historical Perspective*, ed. Huntelmann, Jaser, Roscher, and Weber, 235–284.

Patel, Raj, and Jason W. Moore. 2018. *The History of the World in Seven Cheap Things*. Berkeley: University of California Press.

Phillips, Edward. 1675. *Theatrum Poetarum*. London.

Rogers, Ben. 2003. *Beef and Liberty: Roast Beef, John Bull and the English Nation*. London: Chatto and Windus.

Ross, John J. 2012. *Shakespeare's Tremor and Orwell's Cough: The Medical Lives of Famous Writers*. New York: St. Martin's Press.

Santer, Melvin. 2014. *Confronting Contagion: Our Evolving Understanding of Disease*. New York: Oxford University Press.

Schleifer, Ronald, and Jerry Vannatta. 2013. *The Chief Concern of Medicine: Integrating the Medical Humanities and Narrative Knowledge into Medical Practices*. Ann Arbor: University of Michigan Press.

Schleifer, Ronald, and Jerry Vannatta. 2019. *Literature and Medicine: A Practical and Pedagogical Guide*. London: Palgrave Macmillan.

Slovic, Scott, Vidya Sarveswaran, and Swarnalatha Rangarajan, eds. 2022. *The Bloomsbury Handbook to the Medical-Environmental Humanities*. New York: Bloomsbury Academic.

Spinage, Clive. 2003. *Cattle Plague: A History*. New York: Kluwer Academic/ Plenum Publishers.

Stanyhurst, Richard. 1582. *Thee first foure bookes of Virgil his Aeneis translated intoo English heroical verse*. Leiden: Iohn Pates.

Tanga, Carmen, Marta Remigio, and Joan Viciano. 2022. Transmission of Zoonotic Diseases in the Daily Life of Ancient *Pompeii* and *Herculaneum* (79 CE, Italy): A Review of Animal–Human–Environment Interactions through Biological, Historical and Archaeological Sources. *Animals* 12:213–249.

Thomson, George. 1666. *Loimotamia, or, The pest anatomized*. London: Printed for Nath[aniel] Crouch.

Trevisanto, Siro. 2005. *The Plagues of Egypt: Archaeology, History and Science Look at the Bible*. Piscataway, NJ: Gorgias Press.

Tyrell, James. 1696. *The General History of England, as well Ecclesiastical as Civil: From the Earliest Accounts of Time, to the Reign of his Present Majesty King William III*. London: W. Rogers.

Virgil. 1907. *The Aeneid of Virgil*. Translated by E. Fairfax Taylor. London: J. M. Dent.

Virgil. 1999. *Eclogues, Georgics, Aeneid I–VI*. Translated by H. Rushton Fairclough, Revised by G. P. Goold, 2 vols. Rpt. Cambridge, MA: Harvard University Press.

Wald, Patricia. 2008. *Contagious: Cultures, Carriers, and Outbreak Narrative*. Durham: Duke University Press.

Wilkinson, Lise. 1992. *Animals and Disease: An Introduction to the History of Comparative Medicine*. Cambridge: Cambridge University Press.

Woods, Abigail, Michael Bresalier, Angela Cassidy, and Rachel Mason Dentinger. 2018. *Animals and the Shaping of Modern Medicine: One Health and Its Histories*. London: Palgrave Macmillan.

CHAPTER 2

Dire Plague Creeping: Vermin, *De Mortibus Boum*, and Christian Disease Ecologies

Abstract The centerpiece of this chapter is a forgotten fourth-century poem on cattle plague. Re-edited and republished through the nineteenth century, *Beginning of the Song of St. Severus Endeleichus, the Orator on Deaths of Cattle*, or *De Mortibus Boum* offers an important version of what I call "the bovine elegy," a rural lament for and by farmers grieving their dying oxen, stallions, and cows. Among its several purposes is to theorize, in an age before germ theory, how contagious diseases could spread from region to region, even from country to country, and how disease outbreaks could be resolved. This chapter considers one of the many possibilities of contagion—insects. I examine connections between *De Mortibus Boum* and John Pory's English translation of Leo Africanus's *A geographical Historie of Africa* (1600), with its historical accounts of locust infestation. Pory's translation shares with *De Mortibus Boum* a tendency to divide the world into "Christian" and "Pagan," the latter represented by swarming insects, divine scourges for sinful peoples and nations.

Let Ephah rejoice with Buprestis, the Lord endue us with temperance and humanity, till every cow can have her mate!
Christopher Smart, *Jubliato Agno*

L. Cole, *The Fifth Plague*, Palgrave Studies in Animals and Literature, https://doi.org/10.1007/978-3-031-92793-5_2

"Contagion" during the early modern era floats in a word cloud of associations and phenomena that includes insect infestations, rain, cold, drought, mildews, inspissated air, putrefaction, and divine displeasure.[1] In accounts of murrain, this word cloud sometimes resolves into narrative, into causal explanations, but the causes are always multiple. As Gervase Markham wrote in *Cheape and good husbandry*, "the pestilence or morrain" is bred by "divers occasions," including "rankness of Blood, or Feeding, from corruption of the Air, intemperatenesse of the Weather, inundation or Floods, or the infection of other Cattel" (Markham 1614, 75). Over two centuries later, nineteenth-century physicians and veterinarians remained reluctant to commit to a firm etiology of contagious livestock diseases. The noted veterinarian Robert Jennings cites approvingly his late-eighteenth-century predecessor William Youatt on the indeterminable origin of twenty or so murrain outbreaks between 801, the beginning of the reign of Charlemagne, and the twelfth century. Four of these events, says Youatt, can be traced to "excessive moisture in the air" and "continual rains"; one to "excessive drought and heat"; one to a solar eclipse; one to a comet; and one to "a most unusually stormy winter" (Jennings 1863, 227–28). The causes of thirteen other outbreaks remain unclear, even though, Youatt adds, one may be attributable to a certain Duke of Benevento who, rumor has it, employed people to sprinkle "enchanted powder" over fields to destroy the cattle of his enemies (Jennings, 227–28). Youatt's skepticism about a single cause—even *any* identifiable cause—is typical, both before and after the eighteenth century, of the medical and agricultural texts I study in this chapter.

And rightly so. We now know that cattle plague is comprised of at least three different types of enzootic cattle infections. Rinderpest, caused by a measles-related paramyxovirus, is likely responsible for the first European panzootic and reappeared throughout the eighteenth century. Zoonotic anthrax was also prevalent throughout Europe, and was sometimes accompanied by a third enzootic infection, foot-and-mouth disease, caused by a picornavirus related to human polio (Morens 2003, 886–89). As David Morens has argued, because rinderpest, foot-and-mouth disease, and anthrax were often "coprevalent," they appeared, incorrectly, to be variants of the same disease:

[1]The term "inspissated" means demonically generated "gross vapours raised from earth" which can assume bodily shape. The term is found in Kramer and Sprenger, *The Mallues Malificarum* (1971, 109). See Cole (2016, 34).

> In place of disease specificity—the modern notion that different "causes" (e.g. microorganisms) produce different diseases—observers of the time were more likely to conclude that epizootics and epidemics alike took on different characteristics and exhibited different behaviors—from time to time and place to place—not because of inherently different causes, but under the influence of modifying "local" climactic, environmental, and meteorological cofactors. (888)

The default position, in other words, tended toward what were then called miasmic explanations whose cofactors early modern writers characterized experientially: excessive heat, cold, excessive rain and floods, or drought. Miasmic explanations could include visible atmospheric disruptions or what the noted historian William Robertson called in the eighteenth century "putrid exhalations" that amplify "the malignity of the distempers natural to the climate" (Robertson 1777, 1: 258). In his comprehensive history of animal plagues published in 1871, George Fleming reports on a 1682 murrain on the borders of Italy that subsequently spread to Switzerland; it "seemed to propagate itself in the form of a blue mist," writes one contemporary, which sickened the grazing cattle; most died within "twenty-four hours" of returning home (Fleming 1871, 1: 153–54). Significantly, though, and in ways that complicate any easy resort to miasma theory, the same "blue mist" was described by others as "some volatile insect," or even as a "flying cancer," that traveled "in twenty-four hours, two leagues in length by four miles in breadth" (Fleming 1: 153). Reinforcing Markham's catalogue of plague's "divers occasions," Fleming's history of animal plagues includes over four times as many references to "insects" or "locusts" (85) than to "mist" or "miasma" (7) as proximal causes or possible sources of infection.

Drawing on centuries of literature on animal plagues, this chapter explores the more-than-human complexity of disease discourse between roughly 1500 and 1700. Rather than trying to craft a progressivist history of the early stages of veterinary medicine, I want to focus on causes—environmental, theological, entomological, and even affective—that figured prominently if ambiguously in early accounts of livestock disease during the Little Ice Age. Cattle and oxen were at the center of food and even agricultural labor systems, so the health and productivity of England's herds were critical concerns for the agricultural writers who are discussed in this chapter. The extreme weather events of this period devastated harvests and led to chronic, often dire food shortages; the specters of dearth, disease, famine, and financial ruin haunted almost every farm, village, and town.[2] Although

[2] In Fleming's history, "rain," "cold," and "heat" appear 255 times.

as sources of protein, animals *could* provide some people temporary protection against the risks of climate-related crop failures, Sam White argues persuasively that during the Little Ice Age, European agropastoralism brought with it "major risks" because the "vulnerabilities of domesticate animals came to parallel those of their people" (White 2014, 322).

Dramatizing this shared risk is a mostly forgotten poem about cattle plague, *Beginning of the Song of St. Severus Endeleichus, the Orator on Deaths of Cattle*, hereafter referred to as *De Mortibus Boum* ("On the Deaths of Cattle"). The centerpiece of this chapter, *De Mortibus Boum*, which may be based on a fourth-century text, was popularized (insofar as a Latin text could be popularized) in the sixteenth century and reprinted repeatedly—especially during outbreaks of cattle plague—over the next two hundred years.[3] Although there are earlier and later editions of this poem, the one I use, with elaborate notes by the German scholar Johannes Weitzius (1576–1642), presents thumbnail sketches of several crucial concerns in this study: the inability to cure or even diagnose murrain; shared human-animal suffering; culling as a strategy to contain outbreaks; and the threat posed by insects (particularly, tiny ones called buprestis) as a possible cause of disease.[4] Overall, the poem offers an extended primer on Christian apologetics, focusing on two related ideas: faithlessness as an occasion for God's punishment and faith as offering a kind of prophylactic immunity to ill fortune. While realistically depicting the deadly cattle plague, as in Virgil's *Georgics*, *De Mortibus Boum* dramatizes the limits of animal husbandry and naturalistic knowledge when cattle plague strikes. Markedly polemical in nature, it tries to convert non-Christians to Christianity by representing cattle plague as God's judgment on an evil, blasphemous, or faithless people. At stake in the poem, then, is not simply the health of the herds, but the health of a Christian, as distinct from pagan, nation.

[3] On the textual history of this poem, see Ines Warburg (2015, 185–198). Whether or not *De Mortibus Boum* originated in the fourth century—no such ancient manuscript has been found—according to recent studies of textual and physical evidence, the plague of 569–70 was one of three early medieval major human-bovine pandemics that swept across continental and northwest Europe (Newfield 2015, 1–38).

[4] Severi Endeleichi, *Carmen Bucolicum De Mortibus Boum*, cum *Notis M. Johanis Weitzl ad Jacob Bongarsium Francoforti, Apud Egenolphum Emmelium*, 1612, translated into English by Michael Knierim (see the Appendix). The English translation will be cited hereafter in the text.

Throughout the sixteenth, seventeenth, and (as we will see in later chapters) eighteenth centuries, Christian disease ecologies brought together seemingly disparate elements—weather, cattle plague, and insects—in ways that (1) reinforced Mosaic history, (2) shored up European chauvinism, (3) defined what we would later call disease vectors, (4) determined plague mitigation strategies, and (5) marked entire populations of humans as "healthy" or "diseased." I explore these interlocking discourses by turning later in this chapter to John Pory's English translation of John Leo Africanus's *A geographical historie of Africa* (1600). Drawing heavily on Exodus, Pory's translation demonstrates how ecology, economics, theology, entomology, and agriculture—disciplines now distinguished by subject, method, and scale—were united under the narrative authority of the Plagues of Egypt. I analyze this text at some length because Pory's translation became a touchstone for later writers of natural histories.[5] Both Thomas Moffet in his *The theater of Insects, or Lesser living Creatures* (1634; English trans. 1658) and Thomas Browne in *Pseudodoxia epidemica* (1646) see locusts as God's punishment on human and animal populations in ways that helped map the early modern epidemiological world.[6] Locusts offered for many writers a model of contagion; armies of locusts on the wing helped establish a relationship between infection and infestation. They also could be deployed to explain how infection could travel across geophysical and political boundaries. Although the connection between insects and cattle plague may seem strained to many readers in the twenty-first century, swarming insects, including locusts, played now largely forgotten semiotic and biopolitical roles in Christian disease ecologies and early modern natural histories.[7] Regarded both as a source of putrefaction in theories of miasma and as a possible way of imagining how diseases could be transmitted across vast distances, insects are in many ways the agential but abjected other of Europe's theo-agricultural economies.

[5] On insects, interpretation, and problems of scale, see Campana (2013, 94–113).

[6] Moffet's text was published posthumously in Latin in 1634, and an English translation was published with another posthumous treatise in 1658. See Topsell (1658); Thomas Browne (1646).

[7] Indeed, as Darryl Caterine has argued, during the fifteenth and sixteenth centuries, close to two hundred class-action suits were brought against vermin, mostly insects, in ecclesiastical courts throughout Europe (Caterine 2024, 129–52).

The Limits of Secular Knowledge in *De Mortibus Boum*

De Mortimus Boum belongs within a more-than-human humanist tradition. Petrarch's *On the Remedies of Good and Evil Fortune*, begun in the 1350s, was according to many scholars one of the most influential texts of the Renaissance (Huss 2022, 287–323). The work's "all-encompassing engagement" with the "difficulties of human existence," in the words of Bernhard Huss, is in keeping with Petrarch's intentions: "to establish a community of readers that included nothing less than the *genus humanum* as a whole" (288). Heinrich Steiner's (or Steyner's) illustrated 1532 edition (*Von der Artzney bayder Glück*), first published in German, was rapidly translated into French, German, Catalan, Italian, English, Spanish, Czech, Dutch, Hungarian, and Swedish. It includes 262 woodcuts drawn by an artist—the so-called Petrarch master—whose identity remains unknown.[8] Figure 2.1, below, represents both humans and animals suffering from what viewers easily might interpret as the same disease (Petraca 1532). Entitled by the National Library of Medicine, "Neither Man Nor Animal is Immune to the Plague," this woodcut features a man with an open sore lying in the foreground, surrounded by animals: a dog, a cat, two birds, and a rooster. Two persons, their faces covered against the plague, bear witness to the death throes of another man, lying on the bed, an oozing sore under his left arm. Above him, a woman holds a crying child. A second child, apparently dead, lies at the far left of the image alongside another expired animal, a pony or freakishly small horse. In death as in life, this image suggests both shared suffering and complex cross-species relationships. The posture of the bird on the left of the woodcut, above the outstretched left arm of the dead or dying man, suggests the still-alive bird may have been pecking at diseased and presumably still contagious flesh. The shared susceptibility of these humans and their creatures testifies to the disruptions of zoonotic disease: even if one were to imagine that the two standing, muffled humans survive, their generation has been cut (the dead child), their livelihood is likely gone (the dead pony, the dead dog, the dead rooster, the dead rat-catching cat), and all familial and affectional ties (the old man, the two adults, the dead child, and the crying infant) have been severed irrevocably. Clearly, humanity's

[8] On the problems of identifying the artist, see Huss, 288, note 5. As early as 1620, publishers could no longer identify who had cut the original woodblocks.

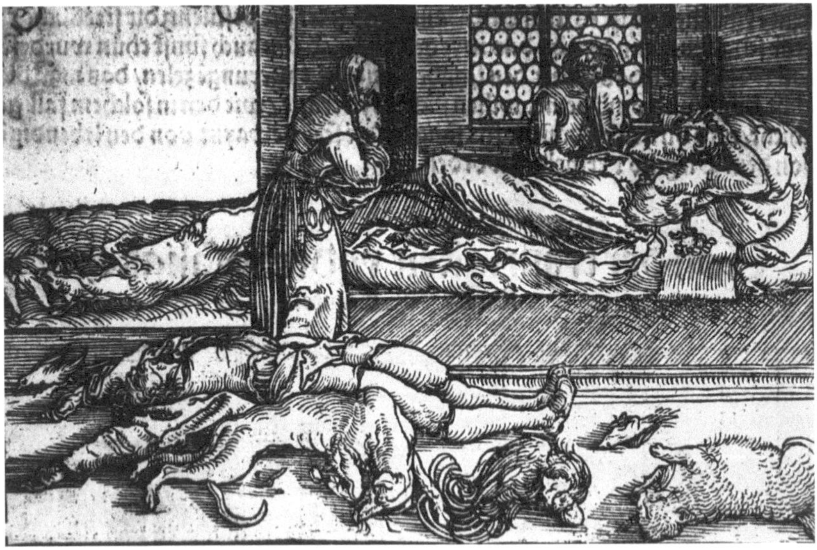

Fig. 2.1 *Von Der Artzney bayder Glück, des guten und wederwertigen* [Neither man nor animal is immune to the plague]. Illustrator Hans Weiditz. Ausberg: Heynrich Steyner, 1532. National Library of Medicine

"bad fortune," at least in the legacy of Petrarchan humanism, includes the fate of nonhuman creatures—both livestock and the domesticated animals of the early modern household. The proximity of the bodies underscores that, epidemiologically and biopolitically, the vulnerabilities of our animals mirror our own.

Although not all editions of Petrarch's *On the Remedies of Good and Evil Fortune* include "Neither man nor animal is immune to the plague," this woodcut represents an all-too-familiar epidemiological reality in the 1500s and after. Germany suffered a "dreadful" murrain in 1499, according to the historian Clive Spinage, followed by a "great mortality" that continued into 1505 (Spinage 2003, 96). Fleming's 1871, more comprehensive, account mentions the 1499 murrain, but also notes vegetable blights, caterpillars, famine, and outbreaks of human disease. "The preceding winter," Fleming writes, had "been so severe as to kill nearly the whole of the brute creation, and the summer was so intensely hot, that trees were set on fire by the heat of the sun" (122). Nor did the following century offer much relief; almost every year brought pestilence to some part of Europe, with many outbreaks affecting cattle, sheep, hogs, horses, alpacas, cats, poultry, and fish (an epizoöty or "distemper") as well as humans (an epidemic). Almost all the mass mortality events of cattle that Fleming catalogues include men and often insects.

> 1505. A very wet summer. Then came the pestilence, which had already lasted several years. It was now more severe amongst the cattle that it had hitherto been, and among men it was none the less so. There was a great invasion of caterpillars in Northern Germany, which destroyed all the foliage.

The next decade (1513–14) brought cattle plague and human dysentery to Italy (apparently motivating Girolamo Fracastoro to begin drafting his foundational tract on contagion); a contagion among sheep in France was followed by a "murrain of kine" so infectious that scavenging dogs and ravens "swelled to death" and "none durst eat beef."[9] In the 1520s, Ireland, Germany, Italy, Switzerland, and France all experienced unpredictable weather, a potentially poisoned food system, and an outbreak of the still-mysterious sweating sickness. The 1530s were characterized by humans and cattle afflicted by "the pest," fluxes, and agues; the following decade brought with it plague all over Europe, along with clouds of red locusts, great rains, and "a great mortality of cattle" (Fleming 134). This list of mid sixteenth-century outbreaks could go on. By 1599, plague "in mankind" had broken out in "various part of the world, but especially in France and Upper Italy," countries that also suffered through "disease in cattle" that killed "thirteen thousand beasts" (Fleming 139).

Reading Fleming's History of Animal Plagues or its predecessor—Noah Webster's *A Brief History of Epidemic and Pestilential Diseases* (1799)—leaves one reeling from the frequency of outbreaks, their multispecies natures, the stark interdependency of humans and animals, and the vulnerability of both to climatic disruptions and various pathogens. My quick overview cannot substitute for the experience of studying Webster's or Fleming's compilations, but it can help establish a historical, affective, and epidemiological context for why it makes sense to devote much of this chapter to a now largely forgotten poem about the death of cattle. As

[9] Girolamo Fracastoro, *De contagione et contagiosis morbis et eorum curatione* (1546). The first version of *De Contagione* was in progress by 1534. See Nutton (1990, 196–234). The outbreaks in France are noted by Fleming, 131.

Petrarch's *On the Remedies of Good and Evil Fortune* makes clear, early modern life was remarkably dangerous for humans and cattle alike.

De Mortimus Boum emerges from the same epidemiological and humanist context as the Petrarch master's morbid woodcut. The 1612 edition is dedicated to Jacob Bongarsius (Jacques Bongars), counselor to recently murdered Henry IV, "the most Christian king of France."[10] Its polemical appeal, like that of *On the Remedies of Good and Evil Fortune*, rests on its depiction of overwhelming despair that multispecies affliction could provoke. *De Mortibus Boum* features a conversation among three characters: Buculus, whose herds have succumbed to plague; Aegon, a sympathetic friend and interlocutor; and the mostly silent Christian Tityrus, who "goes along happily with an intact herd" (ll. 97–100). Aegon asks Buculus at the beginning of the poem, "why is it that you wander alone groaning sadly with heavily downcast eyes? Why do your cheeks run with abundantly flowing tears? Let one who loves you know!" (l. 1–4). Buculus begs to "bury" his "diseased senses in deep silence" but, after Aegon persuades him that conversation helps pain, Buculus confesses that his herds, once so large that cattle "wandering along the rivers would even fill the hollows of the valleys, the plains and the ridges of the mountains," have succumbed to a mysterious and sudden disease (ll. 5–17). The "labor" of his entire life, he laments, has "perished in two days": "So quick is the path for evil things!" (ll. 17–20). Aegon admits to having heard "talk of this dire plague…already creeping upon us" (ll. 21–24). That the plague "creeps," as Weitzius's notes indicate, is almost a classical formula; Weitzius cites several similar usages, including from Lucretius and this, from Virgil's *Georgics*: "Dire contagions creep through the unwary common people."[11] The verb "creep" evokes the growing habit of vines or rhizomes; it also recalls that category of life in the King James Bible deemed neither bird nor beast: "Every beast, every creeping thing, and

[10] Pierre Pithous published what is usually regarded as the authoritative edition in 1586, with reprints in 1590 and 1596. Significant other editions appeared in 1612—the German edition translated here—and in 1772, 1780, 1835, and 1870. I use the 1612 edition in part because of the scholarly apparatus with notes by Johannnis Weitzl, Johann Weitz (1576–1642), and Wolfgang Seber (1573–1634). All quotations are from Michael Knierim's translation of *De Mortibus Boum*, included in the Appendix. I have numbered line groups which are hereafter cited in the text.

[11] See note to line 21 in the Appendix. See Botelho (2023, 2: 132–40).

every fowle" (Genesis 8:19).[12] Verminous in character, allied with "evil" creatures and forces hostile to useful and domesticated animals, this dangerous and mysterious plague kills en masse, blasting within hours the lifelong labor of farmers and cattle herders.

Aegon's next question goes to the heart of Christian apologetics: the limitations of human knowledge and agency. "But," Aegon asks, "since you usually know how to drive away a dangerous death by healthful potions, why didn't you prevent it in advance with your healing hands?" (ll. 25–28). In ways that mirror both Virgil's *Georgics* and early modern husbandry texts, Buculus responds "there are no obvious signs of this fearsome thing. The disease crushes whatever it takes hold of, nor does it allow its victim a period of weakness nor does it suffer any delays, but death comes before illness" (ll. 33–36). *Death comes before illness.* This is the hallmark of murrain as described in contemporary husbandry manuals. These texts, partly devoted to buying, feeding, and fattening cattle, also include myriad remedies for common ailments—worms, colic, fevers, the "bloody flux," or what later would be known as dysentery, and ultimately identified as a bovine coronavirus.[13] Husbandry manuals advocate a variety of treatments based on specific symptoms, usually erring on the side of thoroughness. Significantly, though, the manuals are both brief and markedly pessimistic in discussing the treatments for murrains. In *The boke of husbandry* (1523), which went through multiple editions in the sixteenth century, John Fitzherbert's section on "murren" begins, "And yf it fortune to fall murren amonge thy beastes, as god forbede, there be men ynough can helpe them" – in other words, humans ("men ynough") will never be able to "helpe" the cattle afflicted (Fitzherbert 1523, 35). Believing murrain to "commeth of a rankness of bloudde," Fitzherbert proposes only one possible remedy, and then only if symptoms have not reached the head: wrap a cord around its neck, locate the largest vein, then bleed the animal of a pint or so; once its head swells, though, and the animal's eyes "waxe greate and ronne of water and frothe at the mouthe," the beast is "paste remedy, and wyl dye shortely, and wyll never eate after be sycke" (36). Buculus's inability to keep his cattle alive mirrors the

[12] Genesis 8.19. See also Milton, *Paradise Lost* 7: 452: "Cattel and Creeping things, and Beasts of the Earth." *Paradise Lost, A Poem Written in Ten Books.*

[13] https://www.nadis.org.uk/disease-a-z/cattle/winter-dysentry/, accessed January 27, 2024.

hopelessness described in Fitzherbert and other sixteenth-century husbandry manuals: once symptoms appear, the afflicted animal is doomed.

What distinguishes murrain from other diseases is its "unnatural" quality, the *lack* of symptoms that can be treated. Leonard Mascall emphasizes the difference between animals "diseased naturally" and those "bewitched"—between material diseases that can be cured or allowed to run their course and those that have an occult or theological explanation. If a horse or "other cattell," he writes, "be sicke or diseased naturally," their "griefe" will alter them "litle by litle," and sometimes mend (Mascall 1587, 188). In contrast, death comes "vehemently" to the "bewitched" (188). A "bewitched" horse, according to Mascall, "will eate no meate, because he is so inflamed with such poison… that within xii [twelve] hours many die, or like to die" (188). Mascall then describes the afflicted horse in ways redolent of cattle murrain:

> Some are striken with knobbes and bunches rising in their bodies.... Some with running at their nostrels matter and flegme. Some their eies swelling and hanging out of their head: with flegme and matter roping and running. Some sodainely falle and so die. Some run about in fieldes as they were mad, and drowne themselues in pits and ponds of water, with diuers other infinite waies they vse in bewitching mens cattell, which here I will passe ouer...If it tarry any space, it will be past remedy. (188)

The sheer number of possible symptoms—confusion, lameness, watery eyes, running nostrils, madness, self-destruction—all lead to the inevitable: a quick death. Buculus's afflicted cattle share with Mascall's "bewitched" livestock a sudden and "vehement" end—"death comes before illness."

To reinforce this view of murrain as somehow occult, the next section of *De Mortibus Boum* establishes Buculus as a model, if pagan, farmer. In keeping with the advice of husbandry manuals, he had chosen his oxen well: "I had selected them with what skill I had": they were matched in age—which, according to husbandry manuals, meant one should be slightly older—and both "had the same tameness, the same strength" (ll. 37–39). Because they worked as a team, "their bells sang together," "tinkling in harmony with their twin minds" (ll. 33–36). Mascall lists among the possible causes of murrain "chafing" or working oxen too hard (6–7), but Buculus does not overwork his animals: "The soil was friable, with plenty of moisture," he insists, and the plow therefore turned furrows "with ease" (ll. 41–44). Despite such skill and care, the younger "left ox," recently tamed, "collapses in a sudden fit"; Buculus then unyokes the older one who had always been "healthy and sound" (ll. 45–52). Fearing no more "evils," he is shocked when the latter first shakes "with long spasms" and then bends "down his conquered head" (ll. 49–51). Murrain defies good husbandry practices and strikes without warning, leaving his oxen team "collapsed in the middle of the furrow, conquered by the same death" (ll. 37–40). Without oxen, Buculus cannot plant; without planting he cannot harvest his crops; without this harvest, neither his family nor his domesticated animals can survive the winter.

The poem then turns to a grim series of fatal vignettes, most centering on the death of cows. Although Buculus had hoped for a moment that the cows would be spared—"future fertility" would escape "the present plague"—his illusions, like his oxen team, soon collapse (ll. 57–60). He sees "a young pregnant heifer sinking to the ground," "two souls" perishing "in one body" (ll. 61–64). Another young cow "refusing water, forgetful of grass" wanders "with sinking tendons," then stumbles and shortly sinks "from the manacle of death" (l. 65–68). A calf, who had "just been leaping and weaving playful paths," nursed from his mother, by which he "drew the plague from her diseased udder" (ll. 60–72). Such scenes emphasize the emotional lives of the afflicted animals. The mother of the now-dead calf "saw the hidden eyes of her calf," groaned in "misery," then "sank down and wished to die" (ll. 73–76). Although the author may be accused of anthropomorphizing the cow by granting her suicidal thoughts, this scene captures early modern understandings of the herd: instead of being numbers in a feedlot operation, they appear as members of a larger domestic circle, one in keeping with the Catholicism of the ostensible writer, the fourth-century Endelichius, and most of the poem's early modern editors. The last act of the grieving cow, dying herself, but fearing that the inert calf could be thirsty, is to try to feed him; "dying she moved her udder to the dead one, there just where he lay. *Pietas* flourishes after death" (ll. 77–80). Pietas, highly valued by Romans and often cited as the chief virtue of Aeneas, can be translated as piety, dutifulness, love, or loyalty. But in *De Mortibus Boum*, it takes on Christian overtones: the scene evokes images of the Virgin Mary holding the dead body of Jesus in her arms. Ironically, and tragically, in this instance, the cow's offering of love—her udder—is the source of her calf's death. Such scenes reinforce Erica Fudge's contention that early modern animals were "simultaneously collaborators in husbandry and extraordinary beings constructed by the Almighty for wonder and for use," capable of forming affective, meaningful relationships with each other and their humans (Fudge 2018, 160–161).

Before they die, Buculus's cattle are individualized by their domestic roles. The grieving, piously maternal cow presages the demise of the bull, "the husband and father of the solid herd" who, joyfully pleasing himself, similarly collapses (ll. 81–84). Murrain strips them of pleasure, pain, animation, individuality, rendering them all the same. "Now all the ground is covered in corpses," cries Buculus: "The bodies swell with bulging bellies. Their eyes whiten with bluish clouds. Their legs stiffen with tense feet" (ll. 89–92). Rigor mortis and the early stages of putrefaction render their bodies ripe for carrion-eating scavengers. "Now columns of gloomy ill-omened birds continuously circle around," Buculus continues, as "packs of dogs" enjoy "the cattle's mangled viscera" (ll. 93–96). The poem's quick shift from affective and domestic relations among the cattle to the nightmarish image of feral dogs and vultures feasting on their corpses inverts the normal state of agrotheology, in which humans dine on their purposefully bred and fattened cattle. Instead, the scavenging scene reminds the reader how rapidly the entire system can crash, and how devastating mass mortality events can be, bringing individual and often collective ruin. "Alas!" Buculus cries, "Why don't they eat my own innards as well?" (l. 93–96). If his suicidal ideation seems an overreaction or poetic hyberbole, we need to keep in mind the plight of farmers in parts of twenty-first-century India, where, according to some estimates, crushed by debt, loss of ground water, and environmental degradation, over thirty workers in the agricultural sector die by suicide every day.[14] Indeed, given the contagious, collective consequences of murrain, Aegon is similarly undone: "I am in pain," he cries, "I am crucified, I mourn, I am in grief! My heart is consumed by your losses just as it is consumed by my own!" (ll. 53–56). Aegon's full-bodied commiseration seems intended to stand in for the multiplicity of early modern readers' responses: they should pity dead cattle, empathize with Buculus's grief and his financial losses, and recognize—with horror—that the ground covered in "funerals" likely heralds their own future ruin. Cattle murrains are never merely economic disasters but catastrophes that define the limits of agrotheology.

[14] https://www.cnn.com/2022/03/17/opinions/india-farmer-suicide-agriculture-reform-kaur/index.html, accessed March 2, 2024.

Supernatural Immunity and Small Spiders

Near the end of the poem, Buculus asks Tityrus, who so far has been silent, several questions: why is his the only "intact herd?" what god "snatched you out of these calamities?" why has "the cattle plague that devastated your neighbors…not harmed you?" (ll. 97–99). Seber's note to this line reads that "something of this sort happened long ago in Egypt when the Lord sent a great plague on the domestic animals through Moses," but that meanwhile "not one of the Israelite's animals died."[15] Tityrus's response underscores the poem's biblical interpretation of supernatural immunity:

> The sign, which they say is the cross of the only god worshiped in the big cities, Christ, the glory of the perpetual Divinity, and its only son. This sign, added to the middle of the foreheads of all the herds, was their sure safety. Truly, this is why the god that is powerful in this name is so often called Savior. (ll. 101–112)

In a gesture reminiscent of the prayer of St. Anthony, Tityrus's herd, it turns out, has been blessed because their master is a devout Christian. "Drive away the harmful disease that is raging among the animals," goes one version of the prayer of St. Anthony, "so that, as with justice You punish those who wander from Your paths, so with mercy You may assist them when they have mended their ways."[16] During the Middle Ages and the early modern era, marking crosses on the forehead of cattle was one of many occult prophylactic measures employed to ward off cattle plague. Others were more grotesque, including cutting off the head of a live two-year-old animal and hanging it up in the house, with the eyes facing east (Northern Germany); hiding a skull under the ridge of a house (Northern Europe); or hanging the head of a horse in a stall (Wales) (Spinage, 96).

But unlike these folk practices, marking crosses on cattle's foreheads functioned as a kind of recruiting ritual, seeking, like Tityrus in *De Mortibus Boum*, to turn heathens into Christians. Reporting on this practice in 1757, during England's second great cattle plague, the physician Daniel Layard, in his *Essay on the Nature, Causes, and Cure of the Contagious Distemper among the Horned Cattle in these Kingdoms*, traces

[15] See Seber's note to line 98.

[16] Dachauer 1956, https://www.catholicculture.org/culture/liturgicalyear/prayers/view.cfm?id=1487.

reports of cross marking to Cardinal Baronius, whose 12-volume *Annales Ecclesiastici*, a history of the Church's first twelve centuries, was published between 1588 and 1607. "Cardinal Baronius says, that in the year 376, when the cattle died of the plague all over Europe, *none escaped but such as were marked on the forehead with the sign of the Cros, by which miracle many people were converted to Christianity*" (Layard 1770, 11). For Tityrus, the cross is a powerful symbol, but only a symbol. Although "severe plague immediately fled" (l. 113) from his blessed herds, even without the mark, even without the cross, he maintains, God will offer protection to the faithful: "belief," he says, "is sufficient. Faith alone helps the prayer" (l. 116). The cross, then, functions as a material and symbolic branding of the owner's or herder's faith and signals Christianity's victory over the pagan beliefs of Buculus and Aegon. Their herds devastated, both men readily agree to convert. "If you vouch for these things as true, Tityrus," says Buculus, "I will make no delay, but I will serve the true sacred ways and gladly flee from the old error, for it is empty and deceitful" (ll. 121–124). Aegon concurs: "Include me also in your prosperous plans. For why should I doubt that the same sign that conquers that power of disease should not also be of benefit to human beings in the age without end?" (ll. 121–129). The "intact herd," marked by the cross, stands in for a human community safeguarded by its Christian faith, one where health and prosperity are intertwined states of grace.[17]

Although the Latin text of *De Mortibus Boum* avoids causal explanations for cattle plague in favor of a conversion narrative, a candidate appears in the editorial apparatus. One verse, as we have seen, describes the ground "covered in corpses," the cattle's bodies swollen "with bulging bellies." In annotating this line, Seber writes that swollen bellies are a consequence of "bodies that have been seized by poison taken in with feed," and then quotes Pliny: "'the cattle burst after devouring *buprestis*'." In his note to line 96, Seber goes on to describe buprestis as an "insect . . . similar to the long-footed beetle. It often encounters cattle unobserved in the grass." Sir Thomas Elyot, in the sixteenth century, defines "*Buprestis*" as "a fly lyke to a blacke bytell, but he hath lengar legges, whiche if a beaste

[17] In a note to these lines, Seber takes up the issue of what it means for "cows and other brute animals" to be marked with the Cross, asking rhetorically, "*Does God really care about cows?*" The answer, in his interpretation of the poem, is *yes*. He suggests that "one could fittingly apply 1st Corinthians 9.9 to this," invoking a passage about allowing oxen to eat while plowing, often cited as proof of God's solicitude toward brute creation.

dothe eate, he swelleth, and therwith dyeth" (Elyot 1545, B Ante V, unpaginated). A century later, buprestis would be invoked to explain the symptoms—particularly swelling—that distinguished endemic cattle plague. In his *Theatre of insects, or Lesser living Creatures*, Moffet refers to Pliny and Nicander on buprestis affliction (which he calls *Burncow*, or *Burstcow*), and summarizes the medical relationship in a couplet:

> When cowes or calves are sick, and bellies swell,
> They 'ave eat *Buprestis* keepers know full well. (1000)

Despite the confidence expressed by this couplet, and in keeping with Moffet's devotion to thoroughness, the English translation of his text includes twenty-eight references to buprestis, some of them inconsistent with each other. A late sixteenth century, pan-European text, *Maison Rustique, or The countrey farmer*, translated into English by Richard Surflet in 1616, describes similar effects but in greater detail: "The small beast abiding in the grasse, called of the Latines *Buprestis*, and resembling in some sort the beast which the French men call *Fouillemerde*, if it be eaten of Oxen, Kine, or Horse, as they feed in the meadowes, it so swelleth them as that they burst and die, as we haue obserued in many, in the yere past 1572" (Estienne 1616, 102). In some cases, buprestis is described as a plant or perhaps fungus and, in many others, like Elyot's text, as an insect or beetle. Its ambiguous status as a "beast" or possibly a plant, as a flying insect or a crawling beetle, made it a catch-all explanation in an era when everyone was uncertain about how livestock diseases actually spread. Buprestis had a long life in etiologies of cattle plague, then, because it brought together scattered references from classical and biblical texts and then yoked them to the experience of herders confronted by the loss of their animals.

In his 1646 *Pseudodoxia epidemica*, subtitled *Enquiries into very many received tenents and commonly presumed truths*, Sir Thomas Browne conducted experiments to ascertain the accuracy of accounts he had heard from "Country people" about something in the grass that could poison cattle. Like Moffet, he reasons back from the symptoms "of the sudden death, and swelling of cattell" to possible causes, temporarily zeroing in on the belief among "Country people" who attribute this disease to their livestock licking "Tainct," a tiny red spider (Browne 1646, 177). Knowing that his predecessors, including Galen, Aristotle, and Moffet, identify buprestis or a similar ambiguous entity as a likely source of cattle disease, Browne tried unsuccessfully to sicken dogs, chickens, calves, and horses with "Tainct"; yet he "never could finde the least disturbance ensue" among these animals. Having ruled out small red spiders as a disease vector, he posits that there may be other tiny insects responsible for the "sudden death, and swelling of cattell" (177). The key point for him, though, is more general than locating a specific causal agent: he wants to establish that tiny spiders and insects "are indeed capable of poysoning and destroying creatures" many times their "bulke." To support this contention, he turns to popular European literature on Africa:

> For if as Leo Africanus reporteth, the tenth part of a graine of the poyson of Nubia will dispatch a man in two houres, if the bite of a Viper and sting of a Scorpion, is not conceived to impart so much, if the bite of an Aspe will kill within an houre, yet the impression scarce visible, and the poyson communicated not ponderable, we cannot as impossible reject this way of destruction; or deny the power of death in so narrow a circumscription. (177)

Even the skeptical Browne, then, remains open to the possibility of death by insect, if mostly on principle and by analogy to venomous African snakes.

Browne's inquiries into "many received tenents and commonly presumed truths" offer a kind of differential diagnosis, an experimental effort to distinguish between an innocuous spider and a noxious agent of disease, like Moffet's buprestis. Browne's attempt to validate or rule out the claims of "Country people" emerges from seventeenth-century efforts to describe the etiology of disease. Browne was in good company. In Germany, Browne's contemporary Ludwig Holberg (1585–1654) refers to a hypothesis "which assumes that the plague is caused by small poisonous insects in the air, which kill by their poisonous stinging" (cited in Hünniger 2024, 89). This belief recurs repeatedly throughout the early modern period, even though neither buprestis nor tainct nor, for that matter, cattle disease could be identified definitively. Buprestis is an ideal rhetorical strategy for explaining cattle disease because it evokes, rather than defines; a close cousin to the scourge insects that played such a critical role in Exodus, it *gestures* toward a specific etiology of cattle disease. Although we use the word "insect" in the English translation of *De Mortibus Boum*, the Latin word is "*vermiculus*," which, according to Michael Knierim, might be better rendered "little creepy crawly worm-like thing." The "dire plague creeping" of *De Mortibus Boum* evokes, then, without committing to, an entire world of causal interpretation, one closed off or superseded by the sign of the cross.

Armies of the Lord

The link between verminous things and cattle plague had a long-standing tradition in biblical commentary. As late as 1799, Webster referred to the Exodus account as "the most ancient authentic history now extant" and used it to explain contagious diseases for humans and animals alike (24). Figure 2.2, from the Cologne Bible (1483), depicts at least two plagues, implying by their proximity that the fourth (flies, insects, swarms, vermin) and the fifth are biophysically as well as theologically related.

The domestic animals of the late medieval farm—a horse, sheep, bull, goat, and boar—lie dead or dying, afflicted, it seems, by the flies that hover above them. God's finger pointing to the flies symbolizes his authority—these flies arrive as a providential scourge. Moses gestures with two fingers, perhaps implying a temporal and physical connection between the fourth plague, swarms of insects, and the death of livestock. Although the

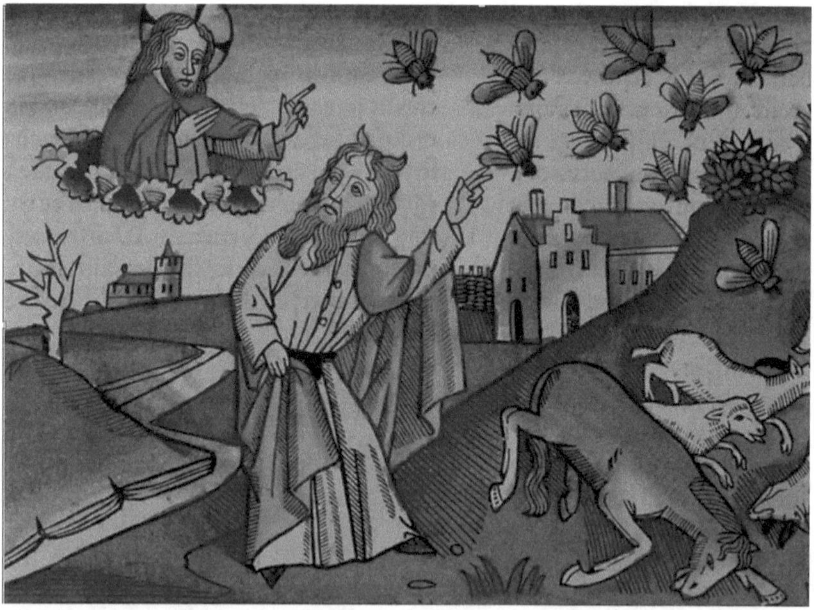

Fig. 2.2 The Plague of Flies, illustration for the German Bible (Nuremberg: Anton Koberger, 1483) with colored illustrations from the Cologne Bible (Heinrich Quenteil, 1479–1480)

victims in this woodcut are Egyptians (although ancient Egypt looks a lot like fifteenth-century Europe), rather than a presumably model farmer like Buculus, *De Mortibus Boum* and the fifth plague rely on a similar structural logic. Insects serve as potential disease vectors and as intermediaries of God's divine justice.

The identification of swarming insects as potential disease vectors persists into the nineteenth century, in part because the microscope brought the miniscule or invisible into the field of vision, and in part because the eighth plague—the plague of locusts—continued to be associated with epidemics. Locusts or locust-like insects were a widely acknowledged source of putrefaction, and putrefaction was believed to be responsible for any number of infectious diseases, including cattle and human plagues.[18] In his history of animal plagues, Fleming includes a short history of fatal locust events. After the eruption of Mt. Etna in B.C. 126, the locusts, having "devoured all vegetation, even to the bark of trees," were driven by a southern gale into the sea and drowned, "after which they were again washed on shore during hot weather, and putrefied there" (18). In this instance and others, locust-induced famine precedes the mass die-off of the insects; they putrefy, and their rotting carcasses become the immediate cause of disease: "The pestilence occasioned by the decomposition of their bodies," Fleming continues, "destroyed more than a million people, and the domestic animals also suffered. The odour was intolerable" (18). Among his ancient sources, Fleming cites the account of St. Jerome in the early Christian era, who describes locust swarms "over the land of Judea" driven out to sea by "the mercy of God," only to end up in "heaps" on the shores, thereby corrupting the air, "and produc[ing] a pestilence both among men and some kinds of animals" (37). In 591, a plague of locusts, presumably from Africa, "eate all the vegetation," then "as usual" were blown into the sea, washed up on the shore, and, putrefying, "killed nearly a million of men and beasts"" (41). A.D. 895–7, according to Fleming, brought "the first recorded invasion of locusts in Britain and Ireland, preceded by bloody rain, followed by a general scarcity, when great mortality of cattle and other animals occurred: the effects lasted thirteen years"

[18] "Locust-like" is a term used to acknowledge ongoing debates about the differences between locusts and grasshoppers. On insect infestation in Ireland and Wales, see Thornton (1996, 37–53), and Cole (2018, 136–155).

(50). In 1091, after killing floods, immense "swarms" of locusts arrived, darkening the sun, and "from their putrefaction next year arose a most desolating plague in man and beast" (64). Although Fleming's compilation is representative rather than complete, he describes clear-cut causal mechanisms: insects—driven by winds, storms, and the hand of God—descend and devastate food stores, then die; their putrefying carcasses poison the air, wreaking epidemiological havoc among already-weakened livestock and people.

Such insect- or vermin-based theories of contagion offered a distinct advantage over either simple theological explanations of divine wrath or theories of miasma as a local, environmental phenomena. Neither of those could explain how disease traveled from one region to another, how a murrain or plague in France, say, could also emerge in England. Insects, by contrast, embody the very idea of the mobility of disease; the insistent linking of locusts to both human and animal epidemics provides commentators and their readers with a means—a "cloud," an "army," a swarm—to visualize disease transmission.[19] In his *Theatre of insects*, Moffet reports that while he was drafting his chapter on locusts he "received news that the Spaniards were sorely afflicted" with swarms of Locusts that "flew like Armies through the skies and darkned the air" (987). In their ability to cover vast distances, locusts embody the inchoate fear that disease and famine can be visited on human communities and their herds of domesticated animals from afar. They offer an authoritative paradigm, grounded in classical, biblical, and natural history, for thinking about how contagion moves from region to region, nation to nation, and sometimes even from continent to continent.

At least through the seventeenth century, most plagues, like those of Exodus, were thought to originate in Africa, and this origin is a significant and overdetermined feature of Christian disease ecology. Admittedly, Europe had its share of insect plagues, including occasional infestations of grasshoppers or locusts. Moffet reports on insect-induced famine events in France in 455, 874, 1337, 1353, and 1374 when a third of the inhabitants died; in 1476 locusts "wasted almost all *Polonia*"; and in 1536 they invaded first Eastern Europe then Germany and Italy, and returned in

[19] For Holberg, Hünniger writes: "'Like flying armies in the air' or a 'gang of predatory birds', insects thus moved from territory to territory, but spared certain areas" (89). For a general account of early modern insects and disease, see Ziegler and Smith (2024, 45–67).

1543, their bodies "forming heaps above a cubit high" (987). Both before and after the early modern period, locust-like insects devastated crops as far north as Wales and Ireland, which also experienced devastating cattle plagues, called in Ireland *mael garbh*.[20] But, for Moffet, as for most of his European contemporaries, Africa is the continent most subject to famine, in no small part because of their locust populations. In *Lesser living Creatures*, he includes a poem about famine-producing insects that "came flying out of Africa":

> —The nurse childe of death,
> Famine was present with her empty veins,
> The poor with hunger starved, their breath
> Was spent; for neither broth nor bread remains:
> Upon their mouthes and guts hunger laid hold,
> They move their chaps, and bite their teeth, not meat,
> Through wrinkled skin their bowels might be told:
> Nothing but skin and bone, they'd nought to eat,
> In stead of belly stood an empty place. (986)

Moffet describes in graphic detail the stakes in the "battle" against what he calls "so cruel an Army," the swarms of locusts that could devastate crops and consequently beggar or starve entire populations. His language is not hyperbolic. A locust swarm may extend from 150 to 400 square miles; 50 million locusts, according to one expert, can eat 100 tons of food every night (Schmetzer 1988). The belief that God sends armies of insects to punish Africans for their paganism was a staple of Christian disease ecology. Those "creatures," writes Moffet, "are not the smallest amongst the Armies of the Lord of hosts, when he pleaseth to punish the sins of men, and to revenge himself on the despisers of his Lawes" (987). This military metaphor was commonplace in characterizing insect swarms. Samuel Purchas, to take only one example, uses almost identical language: we "must conclude that these small creatures have a chief place among Gods Troops and Armies" (Purchas 1657, 201). A century later, in James Thomson's more naturalistic but no less theologically-driven poem, *The Seasons*, plague appears as the "fiercest Child of NEMESIS DIVINE" a "great Destroyer sprung" from "*Ethiopia*'s poison'd Woods,/ From stifled *Cairo*'s Filth, and fetid Fields/ With Locust-Armies putrefying

[20] See Thornton, 37–53, and on cattle plague in Ireland see Lucas (1989) and Slavin (2012, 1239–66).

heap'd."[21] Thomson locates the origin of the plague in Egypt's "fetid Fields," but the carriers are locusts that travel north from "*Ethiopia*'s poison'd Woods," to stifling and filthy Cairo, and then to threaten Europe. Locusts swarm from location to location, devastating crops, corrupting the health of humans and livestock, rendering them, through still mysterious means, susceptible to contagious disease. Even as late as the eighteenth century, locusts serve to connect biblical and epidemiological history in ways earthquakes, droughts, harvest failures, and buprestis by themselves cannot.

History Against the Pagans

It is telling that so many of these European writers, including Thomson, turn to Leo Africanus to target Africa as the source of human and bovine plagues. Christian disease ecology helped map the world spatio-temporally and morally by sorting people into groups partly characterized by agricultural practices and regional diets. If Egypt in Exodus served to link insects to cattle plague, and cattle plague to paganism, texts like Paulus Orosius's *History Against the Pagans* (ca. 417) and Francis Alvarez's *A True Relation of the Lands of Prester John of the Indies* (1540) went one step further, casting the locusts as a God-given judgment on sinful—that is, non-Christian—peoples located in a specific place and time. This abjecting discourse structures John Pory's influential translation of Leo Africanus's *A geographical historie of Africa* (1600), which includes excerpts from both Orosius and Alvarez. Pory's translation contains three accounts of locus infestations; significantly, only one of these is included in Africanus's original text. In Africanus's original, locusts are the last item on a list of animals not generally found in Europe. "[M]onstrous swarmes" of locusts, Africanus writes, "devoure trees, leaves, fruites, and all greene things growing out the earth"; their eggs produce a second generation that continue the feast, thereby "procuring…extreme dearth of corne" (349).[22] Although the biblical tones of the eighth plague of Egypt color this passage, Africanus mitigates the disaster by noting the adaptive measures taken by indigenous peoples: "Howbeit the inhabitants of Arabia deserta, and of Libya, esteeme the comming of these locusts as a fortunate boading:

[21] The quotation is from James Thomson, "Summer," ll. 1043–46.

[22] Pory's translation of Africanus, 349. On Africa and locusts, see Blust, Aldosoro Maya, and Blust (2024, 69–95).

for seething or drying them in the sun, they bruise them to powder, and so eate them" (349). An Andalusian convert from Islam to Christianity (and possibly back again), Africanus had traveled extensively in North Africa. Rarely does he indulge in the extreme denunciations, familiar to many sixteenth-century readers, of African peoples and cultures as "pagan."

In his English translation, however, Pory minimizes any "fortunate" boding, focusing instead on locusts as a source of disease rather than timely nourishment. Significantly, he adds two accounts of locust infestations in his translation and commends their authors: Paulus Orosius is "reverend in regard to the authors antiquitie," he claims, and Alvarez "credible and to be accepted" because he "was a most diligent and faithful eie-witnes of the same" (350). Unlike the descriptions by Africanus, which recognize the power and ingenuity of cultural adaptation, Orosius and Alvarez, Pory suggests, demonstrate how God uses locusts "as a most sharp scourge between times to discipline all the nations of Africa" (958). *History Against the Pagans* tells the story of "an horrible and extraordinarie destruction" visited on Africa. According to Orosius, God sent locusts that devoured corn, bark, and even the wood of the trees, a fitting punishment for the pagans' rejection of Christianity. Although a "violent and sudden winde" bore the locusts aloft and out to the African sea, where they drowned, their "lothsome and putrified carcases" were cast back onto the shore, where "an incredible stinking & infectious smell" brought about a general pestilence, which first killed birds and beasts and then men by the thousands (350). "Never [before] in the time of Christians," Orosius concludes, did a "scourge of locusts" (351) bring such devastation. Paganism itself, in this theological context, becomes a disease vector, drawing God's anger and punishment in the form of a devastating locust infestation and its consequences: rotting corpses, "infectious" air, and a multispecies plague visited on humans and animals.

Alvarez's lengthy description of several locust infestations in India and Africa, also added by Pory, similarly reinforce the presumed prophylactic qualities of the Christian faith. First, Alvarez reports on swarms in India, including one that covered 24 miles, and that made the people "halfe dead for sorrow" (352). In good colonialist fashion, Alvarez claims that the indigenous people implored the Portuguese to help drive off the locust swarms. Alvarez and the Portuguese Ambassador accordingly arranged a procession; they marched through fields of wheat with a crucifix in hand, the Portuguese singing the liturgy and the indigenous people asking, in their language, that God have mercy. Alvarez then excommunicated the locusts.

> I pronounced over [the locusts] a certaine conjuration, which I had about me in writing, having made it that night, requesting, admonishing, and excommunicating them, enjoining them within the space of three howers to depart towards the sea, or to the land of the Moores, or the desert mountaines, and to let the Christians alone: and they not performing this, I summoned and charged the birdes of heaven, the beasts of the earth, and all sorts of tempests, to scatter, destroy, and eate up their bodies: and to this effect, I took a quantitie of locusts, making this admonition to them present, in the behalfe likewise of them absent, and so giving them liberties, I suffered them to depart. (352)

The conjuration, according to Alvarez, successfully drove the locusts out to sea, where a "great cloud" and thunder "met them full in the teeth" (353). After three hours of rain, thousands of locust bodies lay in "mightie heapes" on the shore; the next morning, not one locust could be "found alive upon the earth" (353). Stories of this triumph spread so quickly that, in a different village three days later, the Portuguese were again enjoined to drive out the locusts; they again formed a procession, again read the "admonition," and once again cleared the fields and sky of insect swarms. Pory's embellishment of Africanus therefore transforms the original cultural geography of unknown lands into naked biopolitics: Africa's and South Asia's creatures (both human and nonhuman) become subject to the power of Christian theology through the logics of infestation, excommunication, and extermination. In this respect, locusts underwrite a new physico-theological order: God instructs Christians to rid Africa and India of the insects that serve as both evidence of these regions' need for colonial intervention and as markers of their sins in resisting a divinely sanctioned regime.

The crops and cattle that were destroyed by locusts in "*Ethiopia*'s poison'd Woods" and elsewhere paradoxically served as markers of the prosperity of these cultures. European perceptions of the wealth of Africa, as Rebekah Mitsein argues persuasively, rested on awareness of the continent's political and economic power as well as its natural resources (Mitsein 2022, 1–39). Food, transport, and labor systems in Africa had depended on cattle for millennia; the holiest animals of ancient Egypt were cows and bulls, and cattle may have been present on the continent for the last

10,000 years (Hanotte et al. 2002, 336–339). Africanus mentions cattle eight times in *A geographical historie*, in each case emphasizing their abundance. All lands along the Niger "abound both with cattle and corne"; all Egypt is "exceeding fertile," especially Sahid which excels for "corne, cattle, fowles, and flaxe" (34, 297). Many African cultures also ate more widely and variably than their European counterparts, which made them less reliant on livestock or diminishing stocks of wild game. And because entomophagism, or eating insects, was comparatively common across Africa, it was hardly the chronically starving continent that Moffet represents. Africanus's description of locusts as a "fortunate" boding gestures to a diet born of choice as well as necessity; in parts of Africa, Asia and Australia, insects—nutritious alternatives to beef, pork, and chicken—have been staples for centuries. Globally, as many as 2500 insect species are edible, and Africa is home to over 1000 types.[23] One research team has identified 342 edible insects that have been part of the diets of 94 out of approximately 650 indigenous tribes in India, a practice both acknowledged and maligned in early modern texts (Manna et al. 2022, 329–352).

That most Christian writers in Europe identified Africa with insects rather than cattle is clearly a function of ideologically and climatologically overdetermined discourses. The Puritan James Hart, in his *Klinike, or The diet of the diseased* (1633), justifies his extensive discussion of locust eating from a Christian, proto-colonialist perspective. First, he explains, that attending to "strange and uncoth Diet[s]" (which includes eating dogs, cats, horses, mules, rats, snails, and locusts) enables the reader to "laud and magnifie the great and extraordnarie bountie of our great and gracious God, in affording us such plentie and varietie of good and wholesome food for sustaining these fraile bodies" (Hart 1633, 83). Second, he maintains, that "travellers" forced to be in such places will have to become acquainted with "uncoth" food in order to adapt and survive in alien cultures. Although "uncoth," as a synonym for "foreign" or "strange," does not necessarily imply a harsh moral judgment, Hart uses it in the more derogatory sense of "unpleasant" or "distasteful" (83). Framing *The diet of the diseased* as a fundamental difference between (blessed) Europeans, with their livestock and corn fields, and the rest of the world, Hart makes it clear that in his mind the "diseased" are those outside this agrotheological economy. Because locusts, he claims—"which we commonly call

[23] N. R. Matandirotya et al. (2022: 14823). doi: https://doi.org/10.3390/ijerph192214823. Europeans also ate Insects; see Tigner (2023, 2: 104–21).

Caterpillars"—constitute "ordinary food among many Nations," especially in Africa, indigenous people are marked as always already diseased. God uses locusts to "scourge the inhabitants of hot countries," he insists, along with "the rebellious and stif-necked people of the *Jewes*" (84). Through a complicated tangle of ethnocentrism, Exodus, and scourge logic, Europeanness is defined against the "alien" culinary and social profiles of Jews and pagans.

Despite their seeming differences from cattle, then, creeping and crawling things are critical to the story about cattle plague I want to tell. In classical literature, insects exist alongside earthquakes, cold blasts, infected air, and other phenomena as possible causes of plague, and, in Exodus, they appear as disease vectors for humans and livestock. Within Christian disease ecologies, locusts both help explain how diseases can travel across continents and oceans and can operate as a metonym for contagion proper. I have focused on Africanus, locusts, and diet, however, partly to defamiliarize cattle culture, which is too-readily naturalized in western scholarship. Ferdinand Braudel argued almost fifty years ago that certain civilizations made choices about crops that partially determined their environmental future. "Europe chose wheat," he argues, "which devours the soil and forces it to rest regularly" (Braudel 1977, 11–12). This choice, in turn, "implied and permitted the raising of livestock," so that "Europe has always combined agriculture and animal husbandry. Europe has always been carnivorous" (12). To Braudel's point, I would add another: basing its agricultural and commerce on grass and later grain-fed cattle put pressure on land and labor. As cattle were squeezed into smaller and smaller domestic spaces, or imported from more and more remote regions, the countries of Europe—and many of its colonies—were pretty much guaranteed an epidemiological future punctuated by epizootic and zoonotic diseases. From this perspective, *De Mortibus Boum* is a predictable tragedy within cattle culture, and its scourge logic a working out of Christian disease ecology. The poem, like so many other texts written, translated, and published between 1500 and 1700, treats cattle disease and the health of believers' herds as lynchpins of an agrotheology based on Exodus, even as it scapegoats Egypt as the source and cause, as well as the victim, of cattle plague.

Carrion and Containment

I want to return to *De Mortibus Boum* and to the issue with which I began this chapter: shared vulnerability to an indeterminate disease. In advocating for faith, Tityrus rejects both animal sacrifices and practical measures. "The altar is not wet with any blood," he claims, "nor is the cattle disease repelled by means of slaughter, but simple purification of the soul attains the good hoped for" (v 30).[24] The "wet" or bloody altar is associated with the pagan practice of sacrificing animals to propitiate the gods. By the time this edition appeared in 1612, however, animal sacrifice was no longer a major issue in religious controversies, and propitiating pagan gods or even relying solely on prayers to the Judeo-Christian God had begun to give way to practical advice and legal measures: quarantine the herd, particularly animals that have been exposed to the plague, and kill infected animals to prevent the spread of contagious disease.[25] In this context, Tityrus's warning against trying to repel cattle disease "by means of slaughter" is a little jarring. While husbandry manuals, as we have seen, rarely agree about the nature of medicinal cures for murrain, and rarely express much confidence about their effectiveness, they almost all endorse the idea that culling, or slaughter of the sick and sometimes exposed animals, is one of the only ways to thwart its spread. Less a function of theology than of epidemiology, targeted culling is the *only* practice on which Fitzherbert, Mascall, Markham, and their early modern counterparts on the continent agree.

Fitzherbert's *The boke of husbandry* offers instructions that were repeated with minimal variations over the next few centuries. To prevent the spread of cattle plague, one must skin the dead animal and bury it deep enough to protect the infected corpse from dogs and other scavengers that might contract the infection:

> Than flee him, and make a depe pytte faste by, there as he dyeth, and caste hym in, and couer hym with erthe, that noo dogges may come to the caryen. For as many beastes as feleth the smelle of that caryen, are lykely to be enfecte; and take the skynne, and haue it to the tanners to sell, and bryng it not home, for peryll that may fal. (35)

[24] In his note, Weitzius seems to conflate—or at least fail to distinguish between—what appear to be two different practices, the first a religious one, which he glosses (via Lactantius) as polluting the "altars by pouring out the blood of kine."

[25] But see Hughes (2007) on the displacement of sacrificial death in literary cultures from the early modern period on.

This "peryll" is, of course, the spread of contagion, and, he suggests, communities should warn and seek to protect each other. Out of "greate charytie," people should mount the "bare" or skinned head of the infected animal "vpon a longe pole, and set it in a hedge, faste bounden to a stake, by the hyghe-waye syde, that euerye man, that rydethe or goeth that waye, maye se and knowe by that signe, that there is sycknes of cattell in the towneshyp" (36). Some fifty years later, Mascall's *First booke of cattel* repeats word for word Fitzherbert's advice about burying the infected cattle, but then inserts a suggestion that even to flay the dead cow could be dangerous. Mascall says that he has been "credibly tolde" that some people who "fleade" animals afflicted by murraine "died soone after," as did "he that went with it to the tanner, and the horse that carried it, and the tanner that tanned it": "all these died soone therevppon, which was thought it was by the infection of the stinking skinne, but beeing true, it was a maruellous infection. Wherefore it is thought good of some to burie them whole, for feare of a further inconuenience" (67). In both cases, the carcass is cast as a disease vector, even if the nature of the disease is not fully understood.[26] *De Mortibus Boum*, in sharp contrast, proposes a singularly spiritual solution—"simple purification of the soul"—as a way to prosperity, even as the speakers witness dogs tearing apart the bulging bodies of diseased animals, Fitzherbert's infected "caryen." Whatever the religious force of the poem's argument, its scenes of mass mortality and scavenging more or less guarantee that the plague will spread and wipe out the herds of Buculus's neighbors.

In rejecting practical solutions to plague mitigation, *De Mortibus Boum* underscores a controversy that I trace throughout the rest of this study: different ideas about how "this maruellous infection" should be confronted. If cattle plague, like the plague of locusts, is imagined as divine punishment without any natural remedy—"misfortunate in its pure state," in the words of Foucault—prayer, faith, and exorcism are the only viable responses (Foucault 2004, 31). If cattle plague is imagined as the effect of "bad air"—miasmas and putrefactions—possible responses include a variety of preventive measures, including clean stalls and access to untainted waters. If cattle plague is imagined as a kind of insect infestation, winds, weather, and draining of the swamps play heightened explanatory roles. If plague is thought to be enzootic, or passed from beast to beast, quarantine and culling are obvious, if painful, mitigation measures. Markham (who

[26] See also Harward (1673, 91).

was slightly more optimistic than his predecessors about a "remedie" for murrain) advocates removing and separating sick animals from the rest of the herd: the herder must "deuide them into manie partes" (a kind of bovine social distancing meant to mitigate the spread of contagion), then "separate the whole from the sicke"—quarantine—"for one beast infected will poison all the rest in short time" (7). Once the cattle are divided according to their perceived health status, they must be further separated from other animals: "ye must put them where no other beastes do féede with them, to the end they doe not infect others therein" (7). In practice, all these explanations and strategies tended to overlap, and all play a role, as we shall see, in national trade embargoes and international agreements.

For the exposed or already-infected herd, however, quarantine, culling, and burial offered the most drastic and likely most effective immediate responses to cattle plague. The point of quarantine, culling, and deep burial was deceptively simple: *to stop the motion*, both of the animal and of the contagious agent—the insect, the plague seed, the vermin. All of these responses play roles in Shakespeare's *Merchant of Venice*, the subject of the next chapter, a play set in a hub of the eastern Mediterranean's cattle market. The overtly Christian polemics of *De Mortibus Boum*, with its straightforward scourge politics, its neat division of the world into city and country, Christian and pagan, are recontextualized in Shakespeare's play. His Venice exists in a cosmopolitan realm defined by an intensified international cattle trade and increasingly sophisticated measures to identify, isolate, and contain threats to both the health of valuable livestock and the socioeconomic privileges enjoyed by their owners.

References

Africanus, Leo. 1600. *A geographical historie of Africa*. Translated by Iohn Pory. London: George Bishop.

Blust, Michael, E. M. Aldosoro Maya, and Evangelina Blust. 2024. Insects and Food. In *A Cultural History of Insects in the Renaissance*, ed. Sherilyn G. F. Smith, 69–95. London: Bloomsbury Academic.

Botelho, Keith. 2023. Locomotion: Creeping and Crawling. In *Lesser Living Creatures of the Renaissance*, ed. Keith Botelho and Joseph Campana, vol. 2, 132–140. University Park: Pennsylvania State University Press.

Braudel, Fernand. 1977. *Afterthoughts on Material Civilization and Capitalism*. Translated by Patricia Ranum. Baltimore: Johns Hopkins University Press.

Browne, Thomas. 1646. *Pseudodoxia epidemica, or, Enquiries into very many received tenents and commonly presumed truths.* London: T.H. for E. Dod.
Campana, Joseph C. 2013. The Bee and the Sovereign? Political Entomology and the Problems of Scale. *Shakespeare Studies* 41:94–113.
Caterine, Darryl. 2024. Insects in Mythology and Religion. In *A Cultural History of Insects in the Renaissance*, ed. Sherilyn G. F. Smith, 129–152.
Cole, Lucinda. 2016. *Imperfect Creatures: Vermin, Literature, and the Science of Life 1600–1740.* Ann Arbor: University of Michigan Press.
Cole, Lucinda. 2018. Swift Among the Locusts: Vermin, Infestation, and Natural Philosophy in the Eighteenth Century. In *Animals and Animality in the Literary Field*, ed. Bruce Boehrer, Molly Hand, and Brian Massumi, 136–155. Cambridge: Cambridge University Press.
Elyot, Sir Thomas. 1545. *Bibliotheca Eliotæ Eliotis librarie.* London.
Endeleichi, Severi. 1612. *Carmen Bucolicum De Mortibus Boum, cum Notis M. Johanis Weitzl ad Jacob Bongarsium Francoforti, Apud Egenolphum Emmelium.*
Estienne, Charles. 1616. *Maison Rustique, or The countrey farmer.* Translated by Richard Surflet. London.
Fitzherbert, John. 1523. *The boke of husbandry.* London: Richard Pynson.
Fleming, George. 1871. *Animal Plagues: Their History, Nature, and Prevention.* London: Chapman and Hall.
Foucault, Michel. 2004. *Security, Territory, Population: Lectures at the Collège de France 1977–1978.* Translated by Graham Burchell. New York: Picador.
Fracastoro, Girolamo. 1546. *De contagione et contagiosis morbis et eorum curatione.*
Fudge, Erica. 2018. *Quick Cattle and Dying Wishes: People and Their Animals in Early Modern England.* Ithaca: Cornell University Press.
Hanotte, Olivier, et al. 2002. African Pastoralism: Genetic Imprints of Origins and Migrations. *Science* 296 (5566): 336–339.
Hart, James. 1633. *Klinike, or The diet of the diseased.* London: John Beale.
Harward, Michael. 1673. *The herds-man's mate, Or, A guide for herds-men teaching how to cure all diseases in bulls, oxen, cows and calves.* Dublin: Benjamin Tooke.
Hughes, Derek. 2007. *Culture and Sacrifice: Ritual Death in Literature and Opera.* Chicago: University of Chicago Press.
Hünniger, Dominik. 2024. Bugs, Worms, and Dying Cattle: Multispecies Histories of Cattle Plague Outbreaks in the Long Eighteenth Century. In *Animals and Epidemics: Interspecies Entanglements in Historical Perspective*, ed. Axel C. Hüntelmann, Christian Jaser, Mieke Roscher, and Nadir Weber, 85–94. Köln: Bohlau.
Huss, Bernhard. 2022. A Bestseller for Humankind: The Illustrated 1532 Edition of Petrarch's *De Remediis.* Translated by Martin Bleisteiner and Gabriella Szlazay. In *Petrarchism, Paratexts, Pictures: Petrarca e la Construzione di Comunità Culturali nel Rinascimento*, ed. Bernhard Huss and Francesca Pich, 287–323. Firenze: Cesati.

Jennings, Robert. 1863. *Cattle and Their Diseases.* Philadelphia: John E. Potter.

Kramer, Heinrich, and James Sprenger. 1971. *The Mallues Malificarum of Henirch Kramer and James Sprenger 1486.* Translated by Montague Summers. New York: Dover.

Layard, Daniel Peter. 1770 [1757]. *An Essay on the Nature, Causes, and Cure of the Contagious Distemper among the Horned Cattle in these Kingdoms.* 3rd edition. London: J. and F. Rivington.

Lucas, A. T. 1989. *Cattle in Ancient Ireland.* Kilkenny: Boethius Press.

Manna, Sourav, et al. 2022. The Practice of Entomophagism in India by Indigenous People: Past, Present and Future. In *Indigenous People and Nature: Insights for Social, Ecological, and Technological Sustainability*, ed. Ujay Chatterjee, Mark Everard, and Dinabandhu Mahata, 329–352. Amsterdam: Elsevier.

Markham, Gervase. 1614. *Cheap and good husbandry for the well-ordering of all beasts and fowls, and for the general cure of their diseases.* London: T.S. for Roger Jackson.

Mascall, Leonard. 1587. *The first booke of cattel.* London: Iohn Wolfe.

Matandirotya, N. R., et al. 2022. Edible Insects Consumption in Africa towards Environmental Health and Sustainable Food Systems: A Bibliometric Study. *International Journal of Environmental Research and Public Health* 19 (22): 14823.

Mitsein, Rebekah. 2022. *African Impressions: How African Worldviews Shaped the British Geographical Imagination across the Early Enlightenment.* Charlottesville: University of Virginia Press.

Morens, David M. 2003. Characterizing a 'New' Disease: Epizootic and Epidemic Anthrax, 1769–1780. *American Journal of Public Health* 93 (6): 886–889.

Newfield, Timothy P. 2015. Human–Bovine Plagues in the Early Middle Ages. *The Journal of Interdisciplinary History* 46 (1): 1–38.

Nutton, Vivian. 1990. The Reception of Fracastoro's Theory of Contagion: The Seed That Fell among Thorns? *Osiris* (second series) 6: 196–234.

Petraca, Francesco. 1532. *De Remediis.* Augsburg: Heynrich Steyner.

Purchas, Samuel. 1657. *A Theatre of Politicall Flying-insects.* London: R.I. for Thomas Parkhurst.

Robertson, William. 1777. *History of America*, 2 vols. London: W. Strahan.

Schmetzer, Uli. 1988. 'Worst Locust Plague in History' Threatens Europe. *Chicago Tribune*, May 2. http://articles.chicagotribune.com/1988-05-02/news/8803130590_1_swarms-desert-locust-locust-larvae. Accessed 2 March 2017.

Slavin, Philip. 2012. The Great Bovine Pestilence and its Economic and Environmental Consequences in England and Wales, 1318–50. *Economic History Review* 65 (4): 1239–1266.

Spinage, Clive. 2003. *Cattle Plague: A History.* Amsterdam: Kluwer Academic/Plenum Publishers.

Thomson, James. 1746. *The Seasons*. London: Printed for A. Millar.
Thornton, David E. 1996. Locusts in Ireland? A Problem in the Welsh and Frankish Annals. *Cambrian Medieval Celtic Studies* 31:37–53.
Tigner, Amy L. 2023. Consuming Insects. In *Lesser Living Creatures of the Renaissance*, ed. Keith Botelho and Joseph Campana, vol. 2, 132–140. University Park: Pennsylvania State University Press.
Topsell, Edward. 1658. *The history of four-footed beasts and serpents . . . whereunto is now added, The theater of Insects, or, Lesser living Creatures* . . . by T. Muffet. London: E. Cotes for G. Sawbridge.
Warburg, Ines. 2015. Proposals for the Textual Tradition of the Poem *De Mortibus Boum* by Severus Sanctus Endelechius. *Rheinisches Museum für Philologie* 158:185–198.
Webster, Noah. 1799. *A Brief History of Epidemic and Pestilential Diseases*. Hartford, CT: Hudson and Goodwin.
White, Sam. 2014. Animals, Climate Change, and History. *Environmental History* 18:319–328.
White, Sam. 2017. A Model Disaster: From the Great Ottoman Panzootic to the Cattle Plagues of Early Modern Europe. In *Plague and Contagion in the Islamic Mediterranean*, ed. Nükhet Varlik, 91–116. York: ARC Humanities Press.
Ziegler, Michelle, and Sherilyn G. F. Smith. 2024. Insects and Disease: Unsuspected Agents of Death. In *A Cultural History of Insects in the Renaissance*, ed. Sherilyn G. F. Smith, 45–67. New York: Bloomsbury Academic.

CHAPTER 3

Zoonotic Shakespeare: Merchants and Livestock in Venice

Abstract In ways seldom discussed, Shakespeare's *The Merchant of Venice* provides telling evidence of the global trade in livestock—Venice was the center of the eastern Mediterranean cattle trade—and its concomitant networks of contagion. Building on the work of other scholars working in the early modern period, I reconsider some key passages in the play, many about sheep, in the context of the disease outbreaks that devastated both Italy and England in the sixteenth century. These outbreaks set in motion rigorous protocols adopted by the Venetian Senate for isolating infected animals, quarantining herds, halting cattle shipments, and, in some cases, prophylactically slaughtering herds in danger of being infected. To read Shakespeare—who was, after all, the son of a leather tanner—in light of his knowledge of cattle and the cattle trade is to confront, in unexpected ways, new perspectives on the real and imagined cross-species infections often glossed over by anthropocentric literary interpretations. Central to this chapter, and to the play as a whole, are tensions between Christian pastoral power and growing fears about an amoral, or even immoral, animal trade driven by greed, violence, and exclusion.

A righteous man hath regard for the life of his beast, but the tender mercies of the wicked are cruel.
Proverbs 12:10

L. Cole, *The Fifth Plague*, Palgrave Studies in Animals and Literature, https://doi.org/10.1007/978-3-031-92793-5_3

Shakespeare was the son of a wool merchant and tanner, who whitened and softened animal skins by a technique called whittawing (Schoenbaum 1975, 60). Katherine Duncan-Jones speculates that because his father's profession brought the Shakespeare family into close relationships with butchers, the dramatist had "early and familiar acquaintance with animal skins, both raw and treated," and that many of the plays "allude either to animal slaughter, or to the processing of animal skins, or to both" (Duncan-Jones 2004, 1286, 189). As a tanner, John Shakespeare no doubt would have been directly affected by animal pestilence and the ordinances and practices by which outbreaks were managed. Duncan-Jones includes among William Shakespeare's many references to calves and butchery a host of satirical associations between foolish men and young bovines, but "other mentions," she writes, such as those in *King John*, suggest a "positive obsession" with calves and calf killing (Duncan-Jones 190). In *2 Henry VI*, the King compares, sympathetically, the arrested Duke Humphrey to a calf being brought to slaughter: "as the butcher takes away the calf,/ And binds the wretch, and beats it when it strains/ Bearing it to the bloody slaughter-house;/ Even so, remorseless, have they borne him hence" (3. 1. 210–13).[1] These lines and others like it refer to the practice of driving exhausted cattle from the countryside into the city slaughter-houses and meat markets. For Duncan-Jones, such images "tug at the heart-strings of audiences who…were deeply familiar with the sight of calves being led off to slaughter," a spectacle, she claims, many "early moderns detested" (192). Commenting on the same passage, Ian F. McGinnes details the routes of cattle and other animals driven from small fields outside London to Smithfield through streets carrying their names: Cow Lane, Chick Lane, Cow Cross Line. "Events like this were a daily part of life" in city and country alike (McGinnes 2020, 81). If seemingly anthropomorphic metaphors are a feature of early modern writing, as both McGinnes and Duncan-Jones suggest, it is, in part, because death marches to the slaughterhouse, guilded animal trades, and animal products played a substantial economic role in the lives of many Britons, including Shakespeare's father. The "bloody slaughter-house" was a reality of sixteenth-century life and, as McGinnes emphasizes, Shakespeare was entangled in a vast economic and geographical network that "required its human inhabitants to identify closely with both animals and animal material" (87). His plays are rife with images that speak to the tangible realties of butchering, tanning, and related industries.

[1] Greenblatt et al. (1997, 247). All citations from Shakespeare's plays are from this edition.

This chapter traces some of these modes of human-animal identification—and disidentification—in a period when mass mortalities from livestock disease resonated far beyond those directly connected to the cattle trade. Consequences of animal epidemics and the agricultural, medical, and economic efforts to contain these outbreaks affected farm labor, transportation, the leather industries, and food supplies throughout the sixteenth, seventeenth, and eighteenth centuries. In his *A brief history of epidemic and pestilential diseases* (1799), Noah Webster lists both devastating human afflictions—sweating sickness, spotted fevers, catarrhs, anginas, small pox, measles, and yellow fever—and scores of reported animal plagues beginning in the sixteenth century. In 1514, a fatal illness of cats and "a mortal distemper" struck cattle in England, followed by another mass mortality event in the winter of 1517: "ravens and dogs which fed on their carcases, swelled and died" (152). Citing Girolamo Fracastoro's *De Contagione* (1546), Webster discusses a potential case of cross-species infection in 1530, then describes how 1543 saw "a great mortality among cattel" alongside human plague in Geneva, London, and elsewhere in Europe (154). A murrain of cattle followed a 1580 rodent infestation in Essex and parts of Kent (165). In 1586 "dogs ran mad" in Flanders (166). A "remarkably dry" two years (1598–99) generated "swarms of fleas, gnats, and flies" (169), and "a very mortal distemper" raged among cattle in Italy (170). Clive Spinage, focusing mostly on rinderpest and anthrax, supplements Webster's multispecies list of animal diseases. He recounts a "dreadful" German murrain that occurred between 1499 and 1503, leading some to fear that "pastures had been poisoned" (Spinage 2003, 96). Two British murrains in 1517 and 1523 (also mentioned by Webster) followed an epidemic among sheep, along with an outbreak among both sheep and cattle in Italy. In 1590, herds of oxen died in Italy, and in 1598 rinderpest "erupted over the whole of Germany," which led to a series of sponsored mitigation efforts, including the burning and burying of cattle corpses. This plague spread to upper Italy in 1599, and more than 13,000 cattle died (Spinage 98).

Webster's catalogue and Spinage's history help draw, in broad strokes, the threats posed by periodic cattle plagues and their disruptions to both specific industries (farming, butchering, tanning) and to an urban population that depended on meat and leather. By the time Shakespeare wrote *The Merchant of Venice* in the 1590s, Europe had suffered at least ten major cattle plagues, roughly one a decade, with several reaching Great Britain. Partly in response to these outbreaks and prompted by the increased cultivation of arable land, a new system emerged in the marketing of livestock:

cattle were raised in rural regions (Scotland, Ireland, Hungary) and driven or shipped long distances to slaughterhouses located on the fringes of urban centers (Blanchard 1986, 427–60; Galloway and Murphy 1991, 3–14). Although this international livestock trade ensured the widespread availability of meat in urban centers across Europe, it had a dark and persistent underside: it created epicenters of cattle disease. The practices described in contemporary husbandry manuals—quarantining sick animals, enforced carcass burials, and temporary injunctions against the import or consumption of potentially diseased livestock—suggest that beginning around 1500 both zoonotic and enzootic diseases became an increasingly global problem, one exacerbated by European expansionism and a transnational trade in animals and animal products.[2] Even though Great Britain seems to have been plagued less frequently with diseases like rinderpest than Italy—in part because, until 1666, England imported most of its cattle from a comparatively isolated Ireland—its farmers, butchers, and investors were nevertheless troubled repeatedly by disease outbreaks in cows and sheep, both local and international.

If Shakespeare's works register the reality of doomed animals plodding through London's streets, they also attest to his and his contemporaries' working knowledge of how herds can be both vulnerable to disease and function as possible disease vectors, potentially endangering humans as well. Consider, in this context, the hero's extended plague curse in *Coriolanus.* "All the contagion of the south light on you," the would-be consul Coriolanus rails, targeting Romans who have fled the scene of battle:

> You shames of Rome! You herd of—boils and plagues
> Plaster you o'er, that you may be abhorred
> Farther than seen, and one infect another
> Against the wind a mile! (1.5. 1–5)

This scene of shaming bears significant historical and biopolitical weight. A southerly wind ("all the contagion of the south") presumably brought effluvia and even noxious insects from Africa and consequently was associated with the spread of disease (Cole 2023, 2: 62–82). Given the perceived ability of the wind to carry both odors and disease, a "herd" plagued by "boils" that "plaster" the skin would be "abhorred" before it was seen.

[2] One early example of such regulation occurred in 1598. The Archduke Mathias in Germany ordered the burning and burying of corpses, separation of sick and healthy animals, and prohibitions against throwing bodies into the river. See Spinage (2003, 98).

In his anathema, modeled on the Catholic rhetoric of excommunication, Coriolanus figuratively transforms his soldiers into afflicted cattle, wandering the countryside, shunned because they threaten other populations. He weaponizes zoonotic disease in ways that conjure up a chilling history of mass animal mortalities in the early modern era, along with the human devastation that such murrains provoke.

Earlier in his career, Shakespeare deployed similar language to satiric effect in *Troilus and Cressida*, which Jonathan Gil Harris has called Shakespeare's most "disease-ridden" play (Harris 1998, 4). Ajax and Thersites insult each other in imagery rife with the language of zoonotic disease: the venom-tongued Thersites invokes scab, running boils, the "plague of Greece," horses, dogs, itches, porcupines, witches, scurvy, asses, and "draught-oxen" to characterize Ajax, a "mongrel beef-witted lord" (2.1. 2–12). When the exasperated Ajax starts beating Thersites, the latter curses him with "A red murrain on o' thy jade's tricks" (2.1. 19). Such curses and seemingly offhand insults gesture to a much larger scale of animal disease, registering, arguably, a sensitivity to enzootic and epizootic events, past and present. Although it would be a fool's errand to try to identify specific diseases from these satiric lists, Shakespeare's language conjures up a chain of potential associations. If one tracks Thersites's "plague of Greece" to a possible historical source, the "red murrain" may refer to the rash-like symptoms of an epidemic that struck Athens in 430, described by Thucydides in his *History of the Peloponnesian War*. Epidemiologists and classicists still argue about whether this epidemic was measles, smallpox, typhus, anthrax, or some other zoonotic disease because, depending on how Thucydides's text is translated, a vast number of humans may (or may not) have died alongside sheep (Shrewsbury 1950, 1–25). Within early modern medical literature, "red murrain" also may refer more generally to the color of the pustules or buboes signifying both human and animal disease. Anthrax, significantly, which was often confused with rinderpest, starts with a reddish-brown raised spot; it becomes even redder until the center forms an ulcerated crater with blood-tinged drainage. And while accounts of bubonic plague frequently refer to these pustules as black, depending on the type and nature of disease, pustules could also appear as yellow, purple, or red (Collins 1685). In short, given the witches' brew of animal imagery in Thersites's speech, it may be impossible to pin down "red murrain" to any particular disease, but it is equally difficult to remove "murrain" from its creaturely context, or to collapse it entirely into a metaphor for human bubonic plague.[3]

In the sections that follow, I examine the zoonotic imaginary in Shakespeare's *Merchant of Venice*; resisting the temptation to diagnose medical afflictions posthumously—Michelangelo's arthritis, Shakespeare's possible syphilis, Samuel Johnson's Tourette's syndrome, King George's porphyria—I want to make visible *non*human afflictions. This task requires putting pressure on anthropocentric reading practices that have all but erased the reality of enzootic and zoonotic afflictions recognized and described, however imperfectly, in the fifteenth and sixteenth centuries. Shakespeare, more than once, demonstrates unequivocally his knowledge of such cross-species diseases, as in *The Taming of the Shrew*; Biondello's comic description of Petruchio's "hipp'd" horse is a virtual catalogue of equine afflictions: "possessed with the glanders and like to mose in the chine, troubled with the lampas, infected with the fashions, full of windgalls, sped with spavins, rayed with the yellows, past cure of the fives, stark spoiled with the staggers, begnawn with the bots" (3.2.45–50). Glanders (or farcy) is a bacterial disease. Always known to be highly contagious in herds, by the early nineteenth century it was treated as zoonotic, too (Wilkinson 1992, 122). Windgalls is a soft leg tumor. Staggers (also sometimes known as gid) is caused by the ingestion of a fungal mycotoxin associated with rye grass; the horse's front legs cross over or "plait" when it walks or stands, which leaves the creature unable to eat or drink. This catalogue of equine diseases works comically onstage only if the audience recognizes such afflictions, and so gets the joke.

Yet zoonotic reading is more than compiling a database of diseases and their treatments, or simply tracking down literary references for a history of veterinary medicine. Again and again when we run across litanies of livestock diseases, we confront the problem of figuration: what do these references signify beyond labelling various illnesses? In Shakespeare, any of Biondello's equine diseases can gesture to a complex vocabulary for characterizing humans and their behaviors. The word "giddy," for example, which appears over thirty times in Shakespeare's plays, is associated with

[3] Arguably, the Norton edition does this. Although "jade" is glossed as a "tempermental horse," the editors ignore the string of references to animals and define "murrain" as "a bloody plague." Thersites's line, "A red murrain on o' thy jade's tricks," can then be treated as a general form of swearing, comparable to Caliban's line in *The Tempest*: "The red plague rid you" (I ii 367).

the most typical symptom of gid: its brain infested with a parasite, the animal turns in circles. In Leonard Mascall's view, giddiness is a problem in the blood brought about by an approaching Dog Star—what he calls "canicular daies"—and symptomized by an elevated temperature and "tumbling & leaping without cause"; Mascall also describes a "turning sicknes" shepherds attribute to a "certain smal worme" hidden under the horn which "causeth them to turne as it were round" (Mascall 1587, 229, 230). The shepherd's "worme" may or may not be the tapeworm *Taenia multiceps* that we now know to be responsible for gid in sheep. But it is hardly necessary to bring to this passage visions of a tapeworm tunneling through Petruchio's brain. What makes the image comic is an identification, or disidentification, across the human-animal divide grounded in shared pathologies. When the Widow in *Taming of the Shrew* claims, "He that is giddy thinks the world turns round" (5.2.20), she *both* uses symptoms of a common livestock disease to characterize Petruchio, *and* invokes centuries of everyday knowledge, experienced firsthand by those who worked with livestock. These experiences, collected and contextualized, speak to the cultural as well as scientific and medical value that can be found in late sixteenth-century animal husbandry manuals.

The Merchant of Venice, rife with images of sheep and their ailments, presupposes audiences at least some of whose members can treat distinctions between human and animal disease as porous. As Laurie Shannon argues, "early modern culture is less provincially human than ours," its diversity of creaturely life more "finely articulated," and consequently, she continues, any hard and fast division between the "*the* human" and "*the* animal" is a product of later modernity (Shannon 2013, 8–9). Similarly, any hard and fast division between the figurative and literal easily breaks down. Bruce Boehrer notes that "the sheep, lambs, rams, wethers, and ewes that populated the works of Shakespeare are overwhelmingly of the figurative variety, illustrating with anesthetic regularity a conventional series of concepts: pathetic helplessness, endangered innocence, sacrificial submission, bleating obedience, errant stupidity" (Boehrer 2010, 164). He dubs this combination of biblical and classical references "sheepspeak," one of the idioms that characterizes *The Merchant of Venice*. Yet significantly the play, like many contemporary husbandry manuals, sermons, and art, renders "sheepspeak" biopolitical. Set in the middle of a vulnerable international cattle market, unleashing a complicated pack of animal figures, and gesturing in covert and overt ways to the discourses of contagion, *Merchant* offers a test case in how to read early modern literature from the perspective of a medical posthumanities. By challenging "merely" figural readings of animal disease—or, better, by subsuming figural readings into biopolitical ones—I want to keep open a space for transcorporeal reading practices that do justice to our historical differences from Shakespeare without erasing our shared epidemiological inheritances. Although the twenty-first century may have eliminated once-common diseases like rinderpest—the last few remaining viral samples now confined to high-risk storage facilities—traces of animal disease, zoonotic and enzootic, great plagues and itches, remain embedded, like the tapeworm, in our historical and literary inheritance.

The Meat Market and Pastoral Power

Centuries before *The Merchant of Venice*, merchants from the Hapsburg and Ottoman Empires were organizing cattle drives from the Hungarian plains, through the Balkans and northern Italy, to Venice. In the sixteenth century, Venice was "the hub of a regional cattle trade," according to Karl Appuhn; even though this trade was often disrupted by war and plague, the Hungarian plains "served as one of the principle sources of beef for urban populations" (Appuhn 2010, 270). Annual cattle drives and cattle boats called *manzere* (steer or beef boats) delivered cattle to the island of Lido, Venice's "garbage dump," where cattle and sheep arriving from Croatia or the Hungarian grasslands were pastured to regain weight before being brought to slaughter (Giromani 2004, 3–12). By the end of the seventeenth century the scale of the Venetian cattle trade escalated "dramatically," Appuhn argues; these "denser" connections "between Venice and the Hungarian plains" made beef and sheep more available to urban populations but at the expense of the health of the herds being driven to market (272). Although herds of cattle, as we have seen, are always vulnerable to infection, the increase of international trade in eastern and southern Europe brought with it bovine epidemics that often threatened to become panzootic across national and geographic boundaries. Even in the 1680s, to take only one example, animals throughout northern Italy suffered a respiratory illness that "moved rapidly from one beast to the next," provoking quarantines of animals and farms; by 1748, measures to control cattle plague included temporary halts to commerce and border patrols to enforce strict quarantines (Appuhn, 279). During an outbreak in Fruili, a military governor of Venice, trying to prevent live cargo from being smuggled over the border from Austria, deployed eight boats with clear orders:

"shoot in sight and shoot to kill" (268). During times of severe outbreaks, quarantines became militarized operations.

Prior to the eighteenth century, records of such epidemiological emergencies in Italy are less detailed but not impossible to find. Lise Wilkinson notes "extensive outbreaks of cattle disease in Italy" during the first half of the sixteenth century, probably a combination of rinderpest and foot and mouth disease, presenting simultaneously (Wilkinson 1980, 820). Girolamo Fracastoro describes one such outbreak in *De Contagione et contagiosis morbis* (*On Contagion and Contagious Diseases*): "at first the cattle abstained from food, for no manifest reason," but pustules discovered in the mouths of affected cattle spread to their feet. "The Infected animal had to be removed at once from the herd, or the whole herd became infected" (cited in Spinage, 98). We have already seen that Webster describes a 1530 plague in Italy killing not only "the wretched cattle, but nearly the whole of the unhappy flocks of sheep"; around this time, writes Spinage, people in Padua and Venice, after eating diseased cattle flesh imported from Hungary, were "afflicted" by an "epidemic dysentery" (35). Shortly thereafter, the Council of Venice temporarily "forbade the distribution" of beef and veal, and butter, milk, or cheese from any animal that had been identified as diseased "under penalty of death" (97). Only mutton was considered safe enough to eat. A similar outbreak—this one in oxen—occurred in 1590, when the Council of Venice once again outlawed beef, cheese, butter, and milk (97). The initial staging of *The Merchant of Venice* coincided with "years of starvation over much of northern Europe," made worse, in 1598, when rinderpest erupted in Germany, then spread to Italy where 13,000 cattle died. When human dysentery followed, the Venetian state ordered the destruction of infected animals. The plague nevertheless moved on to France where, in 1604, the health department in Lyon commanded that any cattle intended for slaughter be inspected by "a master butcher in the presence of a commissioner of health" and that infected bodies be buried two meters deep and covered with quicklime (98).

Sixteenth-century British animal husbandry texts were deeply keyed into the potentially damaging effects of a growing commercial meat market that could exacerbate the consequences of already-common diseases. Mascall's *The first booke of cattell* (1587), written in the midst of these early epizootics, emphasizes in its prologue that "diseased cattell, of wealthie yeoman, and other poore men sometimes have all perished" impoverishing the whole parish (a2r). He reinforces this cautionary tale in the poetic preface to the reader that follows, warning farmers and landowners against increasing the size of their "flocke[s]" without knowing how to attend to diseases; lacking such knowledge, Mascall warns, a "man that is full rich in beasts" may "soon loose them all" (a4v). The ever-present threat of disease, he contends, is exacerbated when one strives for individual profit instead of promoting the collective good—what he calls "the benefit of the common wealth." Instead of breeding recklessly, he insists, the husbandman should "save" members of the flock who already exist. "Therefore in this I councell thee," he writes:

> Seeke first to helpe disease:
> As great a praise to him that saves,
> As he that can increase. (a4v)

Mascall's practical advice, then, is framed by the belief that raising animals for profit must be balanced by efforts to mitigate disease. He is hardly alone in condemning the consequences of treating livestock as cash commodities. As Edward Topsell writes in his posthumously published *Historie of foure-footed beastes and serpents* (1658), rampant breeding practices, without regard for what he calls "mercy," are all too typical of profit-driven commercial husbandry. "I am sorry that our times are so far poysoned with covetousnesse," he writes, "that there is no regard of God, man, or beast, but onely for profit and commodity: for as for the service of God we see that the common deuotion of men, and practise of their Religion, is founded upon a meer hope that therfore God wil better prosper them in worldly affairs" (481–482). These husbandry texts emphasize the conflict between profit and the public good at stake in the commercial meat market. The "good" includes the health of the herds on which Mascall's and Topsell's readers depend. The cattle trade, in this respect, involves three related, knowledge-based practices: what we would now call veterinary medicine, the maintenance of the agricultural and pastoral socioeconomic order, and the communal adherence to religious principles—principles that "covetousnesse" threatens to take apart at the seams.

One way to understand the interplay of these three registers is to consider Shakespeare's *Merchant* in the context of what Michel Foucault calls "pastoral power" (Foucault 2007, 129). Christianity, he argues, brought not only a new code of ethics, but new power relations. Pastoral power is "entirely defined by its beneficence; its only raison d'etre is doing good … in order to do good," and therefore its ethics are salvation or safety oriented (*salut*) rather than politically oriented. Because the French word *salut* means both salvation and safety, "salvation-oriented" takes on meanings closely related to individual and collective health, including matters such as security, protection against accidents, and medical interventions. In this respect, pastoral power must be "exercised on a multiplicity rather than on a territory," Foucault argues, and yet, like the power a shepherd exercises over the flock, pastoral power is "individualizing": "it is true that the shepherd directs the whole flock, but he can only really direct it insofar as not a single sheep escapes him" (172, 129). This "paradoxically distributive" structure of the Christian pastorate means that "the salvation of a single sheep calls for as much care from the pastor as does the whole flock": every ailing and wandered sheep calls on the shepherd to "suspend all his other responsibilities and occupations, abandon the flock, and try to bring it back" (226). Yet paradoxically the "necessity of saving the whole entails, if necessary, accepting the sacrifice of a sheep that could compromise the whole" (226). The diseased sheep embodies the shepherd's dilemma. Should he retrieve the ailing sheep and try to effect a cure? Or, because the disease is contagious, should he sacrifice a sheep that could "compromise the whole"? While modeled on the pastor's relationship to his congregation—which was itself modeled on the shepherd's relationship to his sheep—pastoral power involves not just the clergy but any number of actors distributed throughout the social body. These actors, I suggest, include writers such as Fitzherbert, Mascall, and Topsell, for whom the shepherd tending to his flock is far more than a religious truism; pastoral responsibility is essential to the community's food security and economic stability.

In sixteenth-century husbandry manuals, the complex relations that Foucault describes as pastoral power include obligations that were assumed, implicitly and explicitly, by landowners, farmers, drovers, and shepherds. To attend to the health of the herd or flock and to try to cure or contain the animals' diseases necessarily individualized them for the sake of a greater good. Topsell defends his project by both moral and social appeals to those involved in the livestock trade. He invokes "the dignitie and honourable account which the greatest men of the world in former times haue made of Sheep," in an effort to convert profit-seeking into principled duty:

> and thereby I would incite and stir you up, if it were but one noble spirited learned man, which is furnished with wit, means, and opportunity, to dive

> and pierce into the secrets of English Sheep, and Shepherds, and to manifest unto the world the best, and most approoued meanes and medicines, for the propulsing and driuing away of all manner of diseases from those innocent profitable beasts, and for their conservation in all manner of health and welfare. (481)

Not surprisingly, Topsell's descriptions of sheep, their diseases, and recipes for treatments take on the tone of a manifesto, or perhaps an impassioned sermon, familiar genres for voicing the imperatives of pastoral power. In a long aside on the history of dietary laws, he chastises his country-people for failing to value sheep simply because they are "Gods creatures," and instead caring for them only to the extent they are "profitable and serviceable for the necessities of men"—that is "for their fleeces and flesh" (482). He enjoins his readers not only to open their hearts but to take up their pens: "If you have any compassion," he continues, "learne how to helpe their miseries, and publish them for the general benefite, for he cannot be good which is not merciful unto a beast, and that mercy doth easily die which growth but in one heart of one mortall man" (482). If such passages indicate the importance of wool to the British economy, they also remind us that sheep were critical for "fleeces" *and* "flesh," for wool *and* meat. Sheep, then, can elicit Christian virtues of "compassion" and "mercy," which serve as checks on temptation to succumb to reckless breeding and indifferent shepherding in the name of profit.

Pastoral power and the livestock trade meet in *The Merchant of Venice*. Shakespeare reminds his audience at several points about Venice's status as an important center of the livestock trade. His characters are knowledgeable about, and at times even preoccupied by, the price of meat in an economy driven by imported supply and urban demand. When Shylock's daughter Jessica converts to Christianity, Lancelot jokes, "This making of Christians will raise the price of hogs. If we grow all to be pork-eaters we shall not shortly have a rasher on the coals for money" (3.5.19–21). Clearly this is intended as a comic comment on the stakes in the play for a city-state that depends on a vibrant international trade in livestock. In Act Four, however, after Shylock has demanded his "pound of flesh" from Antonio, tensions between pastoral power and a potentially immoral—or amoral—trade play out in particularly dramatic fashion. After describing Shylock to the assembled Christians as "an inhuman wretch,/ Uncapable of pity, void and empty/ From any dram of mercy" (4.1.4–6), the Duke marks him as one who values profit over community:

> Shylock, the world thinks, and I think so too,
> That thou but leadest this fashion of thy malice
> To the last hour of act, and then, 'tis thought,
> Thou'lt show thy mercy and remorse more strange
> Than is thy strange apparent cruelty. (4.1.18–22)

Regardless of the pity audience members might feel for Antonio or the horror and revulsion they might experience toward the Jewish outsider, the Duke's two speeches already have been overdetermined by Antonio's bleak assessment of his situation and the consequences that he and the other characters anticipate from the Duke's intervention to preserve his life. The bond, no matter how outrageous and "inhuman" it may seem, rests on the assumption that trade, rather than "compassion" and "mercie," lies at the heart of Venice's moral, economic, and legal existence:

> The Duke cannot deny the course of law,
> For the commodity that strangers have
> With us in Venice, if it be denied,
> Will much impeach the justice of the state,
> Since that the trade and profit of the city
> Consisteth of all nations. (3.3.29–34)

Antonio assumes that "justice" is a function of "trade and profit," driven by "strangers," and that denying Shylock's cruel and absurd bond will compromise Venice's economy. The "commodity," of course, includes the sheep and cattle that feed the urban population, and, in one sense, the mercantile logic that drives the Duke and Antonio is reminiscent of the logic of "couetousnesse" that Topsell decries. In scapegoating Shylock, the Jewish moneylender and "stranger" for the economic values that shape "justice" and morality in Venice, the play points to the grim contradictions of an agrotheology embedded in the ideology of international trade.

The title page of every early edition of *The Merchant of Venice* advertises Shylock's "extreme cruelty…in cutting a just pound of [Antonio's] flesh," removing Shylock from the Christian ethos of pastoral power, a banishment cemented by his forced profession as money-lender. His distance from a pastoral ethics of care is both made manifest and occluded in the story of Laban's sheep. While negotiating for Antonio's pound of flesh, Shylock recounts the Old Testament story of how Jacob, a "skillful" shepherd and Laban's nephew, used peeled "wands" during copulation in order to induce "parti-colored" lambs that, by mutual agreement, would fall to Jacob's lot (Genesis 30: 25–43). This tale also appears in Topsell, who does not find it "incredible" that these sticks should change the color of water, and that "diverse colours laid before Sheep at the time of their carnal copulation" should produce lambs of different colors, "for such is the force of a natural impression" (470).[4] In *Merchant*, though, the account of Laban's sheep serves primarily to expose Shylock's arrogant greed. As other critics have pointed out, his interpretation of the story is so economically overdetermined, his flock already marked for profit, that the lines among sheep and the fleece and meat markets become blurred. Is "your gold and silver ewes and rams?" asks Antonio, to which Shylock responds, "I cannot tell: I make it breed so fast" (1. 3. 191–92). His answer is less confession than self-congratulation, a boast about interest that, in retrospect, becomes deeply ironic. Despite his arrogant celebration of profit, he ultimately loses both his money and his "ewe" Jessica to a Christian "ram."

In some ways, Shakespeare's sheep imagery seems to anticipate the ideology of the seventeenth- and eighteenth-century georgic, which Boehrer explains succinctly: "Given that British sheep produce the British wool that produces the British economy that produces the British empire, we should not be surprised to find sheep involved" in international trade (2010, 177). The trade in sheep, though, is always a trade in fleece *and* flesh, as both Shakespeare's play and the husbandry manuals remind us. In this respect, what makes the exchange between Antonio and Shylock so telling is less an imperial attachment to wool than the formative operations of a pastoral biopolitics that precedes the extension of the British empire and that emphasizes the relationship between humans and sheep. Julian Yates's precise term for this relationship is "coeval multiplicities": "'Sheep' and not sheep 'humans' become each other's measure and mirror" in ways neither anthropomorphic nor reciprocally zoomorphic but associated "according to a set of figural possibilities" generated by pastoral power (Yates 2017, 205). These figural possibilities are deeply embedded in the Jewish taboo against pork evoked by Lancelot in Act Three and by Shylock,

[4] In ways that prefigure Jessica's fate in *Merchant*, Topsell continues: "for such is the force of a naturall impression, as we reade in stories, that faire women by the sight of Blacka|mores, haue conceaued and brought forth blacke children, and on the contrary, blacke and deformed women, haue conceaued faire and beautifull children; whereof there could be no other reason giuen in nature, but their onely cogitaton of and vpon faire beautifull men, or blacke and deformed Moores, at the time of their carnall copulation" (606). See Hirota 2017 for a thorough reading of the parti-colored lambs.

earlier in the play, who refuses to eat dinner with Antonio because he does not want "to smell pork" (1.3.28). The logic underlying Jewish dietary restrictions, frequently attributed to the "unclean" scavenging of voracious hogs, invokes a biopolitics that, like the Christian pastoral power described by Foucault, is haunted by the specters of disease and death. The susceptibility of sheep and humans, in other words, is the *pre-condition* of pastoral power and the values and assumptions it engenders. The logic of "sheepspeak," in this respect, depends on the need to protect the flock by seeking to preserve the individual, even when that individual, like Shylock, must be coerced into turning from a ravenous wolf, an "inhuman wretch," into a bleating lamb.

This imperative of pastoral care, however, always entails a recognition of shared vulnerability and the potential sacrifice of the straying sheep to safeguard the health of the flock. "Naturalists," writes the theologian James Woode in *Sheperdy spiritualiz'd or, The improvement of a shepherd's life to soul-advantage,* claim that "no Creature is more subject to diseases than, an Horse, and a Sheep; and this last has many Male-affections, by which it is much damnified" (Woode 1680, 132). In a list that rivals some of Topsell's or Mascall's, he includes among these "Male-affections" (malefactions) "worms by taint" that breed in their feet—probably foot and mouth disease; "Feavers"; and infirmities of the head, such as gid, which "make them go staggering like a Drunken-man" (132). That this description of diseases and disease vectors appears in a sermon, rather than in a husbandry manual, attests to the moral as well as epidemiological equivalence of sheep and humans. In this regard, sheepspeak destabilizes both the identification of the animal as a nonhuman other and the ideology that appropriates sheep as mere figurations of an anthropocentric biopolitics.

A Tainted Wether

Scab had a special place within the agrotheology of sixteenth- and seventeenth-century commentators on animal plagues. Also called "itch," scab according to Gervase Markham is the "most common" disease among sheep, probably caused by "raynie and wet weather," "recognizeable by a white filthy scurfe sticking vpon their skins" (Markham 1614, 71). The "itch," we now know, is caused by a mite called *Psoreptis ovis* and spreads from sheep to sheep by head-butting and rubbing as they try to scratch themselves; in the early modern period, it was sometimes regarded as a "taint" of the blood, "being of a running and infectious nature; spreading itself from one part of the Sheep to another, and from one Sheep to another running over the Flock" (71). Both common and highly contagious, scab gave rise to literary, religious, and husbandry memes about itching. According to Topsell, "This disease the *French* men call *Letac*, and of all other it is one of the most contagious, for our *English* proverb justifieth, one scabbed Sheep infecteth a whole flock" (475). The naturalist John Ray later included the same adage in his late seventeenth-century *Collection of English Proverbs*; tracing it back to Juvenal's Satires, he uses the economically-inflected verb "marr" (1678, 199).

Scab shows up so often in theological as well as naturalist texts because—however contagious—it could be cured through affective ministry. Psalm 23 begins "The Lord is my shepherd" and lists a number of sheep-herding tasks, including "You anoint my head with oil" (Psalm 23:5). As Karen Raber argues in a different context, "before the invention of sheep dip, sheep also required the application of ointments and tars to treat for flies and scab, a task the shepherd had to perform by hand, asking each individual sheep and anointing its coat segment by segment" (Raber 2013, 166). It is this sense of "anointing" that underwrites the analogy in Psalm 23 between divine shepherding of errant humans and sheep-herding activities: "he anoints my head with oil."[5] When Thersites in *Troilus and Cressida* says, "I wouldst thou didst itch from head to foot...and I had the scratching of thee, I would make thee the loathsomest scab in Greece," his curse inverts the practices of good shepherding (2.1. 882). Rather than applying the soothing or anti-parasitical oils of pastoral power, Thersites imagines exacerbating Ajax's itch, torturing him into a painful and infectious ("loathsomest") state. Both the curse and the cure, though, rely on the logic of pastoral power, the extension of the relationship between a shepherd and the flock into the realm of a reimagined Homeric war.

Within the context of the "paradoxically distributive" nature of pastoral power, Antonio's abject self-description is the most intriguing part of *Merchant*. At the trial, as Antonio patiently awaits Shylock's knife, he pleads with Bassanio to let the covenant play itself out: "I am a tainted wether of the flock," he claims,

[5] See also the hero's first lines to the plebians in *Coriolanus:* "What's the matter, you dissentious rogues,/ That, rubbing the poor itch of your opinion,/ Make yourselves scabs?" (1. 1. 152–54).

Meetest for death: the weakest kind of fruit
Drops earliest to the ground; and so let me
You cannot better be employ'd, Bassanio,
Than to live still and write mine epitaph. (4.1. 116–20)

Antonio's self-characterization as a "wether" marks him as a sacrificial scapegoat necessary to the well-managed flock and its selective breeding practices. In the sixteenth century, this management included mass castration, sometimes up to 70% of the males. The "weather-sheepe," Topsell insists, differs from the ram anatomically only in "one property" or "defect," for "he is not fit for generation" (494). By virtue of his castration, the wether is treated as a solitary animal. This "Eunuch among beasts," in Topsell's language, is forsaken by the "Ewes" and the "Rams cannot endure him"; his only real company are the lambs, who "follow him" (494). Gelding is paradoxical, then, in that it increases rather than decreases the animal's potential for leadership. Unlike the "warlike" rams (491) who are prone to rutting and fighting, "weather-sheepe" keep the flock moving. Outfitted with a bell, the lead wether alerts the shepherd to the movements of the flock, which is the source of the term "bellwether," first coined in the sixteenth century. In *As You Like It*, Touchstone, the court fool, accuses the old shepherd Corin of misunderstanding this flock order. "That is another simple sin in you," he claims, "to bring the ewes and the rams together, and to offer to get your living by the copulation of cattle; to be bawd to a bell-wether, and to betray a she-lamb of a twelvemonth to crooked-pated, old, cuckoldly ram, out of all reasonable match" (3.2. 77–80). The thrust of Touchstone's insult is not the "bell-wether's" deficiencies, but Corin's presumed failure to implement selective breeding practices. In contrast to Corin, Antonio-the-wether occupies a complicated subject position in *The Merchant of Venice*; sacrificing his own security, his risky borrowing from Shylock ensures the healthy breeding of the flock in Portia—the "fulsome ewe" who promises Bassanio the "full sum of me" (1.3.82)—and Bassanio, a Jason chasing the Golden Fleece. Antonio himself, however, does not participate in the pleasures of copulation and generation.

At the same time, Antonio's identification as "*tainted* wether of the flock" implies a different kind of sacrifice. Shakespeare elsewhere uses the word "taint" or "attaint" to indicate a broad moral, physical, and even political affliction or a general sense of weakness and decay, a frailty also captured in Antonio's comparison to the "weakest kind of fruit."[6] Coupled with "meetest for death," though, the line underscores a hard truth of husbandry manuals, which often cite "the counsel of Antiphanes": "That is to kill those Sheep from whom you can never expect any more profit by their Lambs, Milk, Cheese, or Fleeces" (474). In addition to facilitating mating practices (two years old for ewes, three to five for rams), the second major duty of the shepherd, according to Topsell, "must be to pick and cull out the aged and the sick Sheep every year, and that in the Autumn or Winter time, lest they die and infect their fellows, or lest that the whole flock go to decay for want of renewing and substitution of others" (474). Implied in the space between "tainted" and "meetest for death," then, is the logic of culling, the violence that guarantees the health and continued productivity of the flock. Implied, in other words, is a necropolitics, a logic of strategic killing or letting die, common both to "good shepherding" and to the unsentimental management of contagious disease.

The nature of Antonio's "taint" is never made explicit. Both Antonio's sense of solitude and what he calls his "want-wit sadness" hover over this play from its opening lines; unlike his companions, Salanio and Salarino, who try to diagnose his condition as either the effect of anxiety or love, Antonio insists that the origins of his melancholy are mysterious, and possibly contagious: "I know not why I am so sad…But how I/ Caught it, found it, or came by it,/ What stuff 'tis made of, whereof it is born/ I am to learn" (1.1.1–7). Antonio's sadness is in keeping with the character of the wether. Topsell refers to Plautus on the "weather sheep" as "the most foolish of all other, a coward, and without courage…a mad dotish fellow" (495). The OED cites Topsell's description as its first example of "dotish," defined in the dictionary as "Foolish, stupid, silly, lacking sense or judgment; having one's mental faculty impaired, esp. by old age." Although Shakespeare does not use the word "dotish," in several places he deploys "dote" to signify a mismatched love, especially in terms of age, sometimes in terms of species. In *Venus and Adonis*, for example, Shakespeare writes,

[6] That reading of "tainted" as diseased livestock may seem too literal because elsewhere Shakespeare uses the word metaphorically. In *Henry VIII*, Gardiner refers to a "contagious sickness," a "general taint of the whole state" in "upper Germany," alluding to the 1524 Peasants' Revolt in Saxony, supported by the Protestant clergy (5. 2. 62–4). In *Twelfth Night*, it refers to vices: Viola claims, "I hate ingratitude more in a man/ Than lying, vainess, babbling, drunkenness/ Or any taint of vice whose strong corruption/ Inhabits our frail blood" (3.4. 319–22).

"how love makes young man thrall and old men dote" (859–61). The term always implies desire, but often a desire connected—as in Plautus's definition of the "foolish" wether—with folly and even temporary madness. Oberon in *A Midsummer Night's Dream* uses love-in-idleness to make Titania fall in love with Bottom: "The juice of it on sleeping eyelids laid/ Will make or man or woman madly dote/ On the next live creature it sees" (2.1. 542–45). Even though Antonio denies that his condition derives from his obsessive and mismatched love for Bassanio, his self-described status as a wether reinforces this reading.

Pastoral biopolitics are, however, most clearly at work in Antonio's rescue by Portia who, in his words, has "given me life and living" (5.1.285). Although "life" may be taken literally—a cross-dressing Portia saves him from the knife—and "living" refers to his mercantile ventures, this scene recalls, in a secular mode, Jesus's words to the Jews who demand that Christ declare himself the son of God. "But ye believe not, because ye are not of my sheep": "My sheep hear my voice, and I know them, and they follow me: And I give unto them eternal life" (King James Bible, John 10: 27–28). In the Bible, Jesus is stoned; in *Merchant*, thanks to Portia, the old and tainted wether escapes the sacrificial violence threatened by Shylock in ways that resonate with Topsell's call for "compassion": "he cannot be good which is not merciful unto a beast, and that mercy doth easily die which groweth but in one heart of one mortall man" (482). Shylock, too, is shown a kind of solicitude, even though he gives none. That Shylock is forced to become a Christian—that is, forced into the flock—closes off the pastoral drama in ways satisfying to Christian community. Shylock's "conversion," in other words, like Antonio's renewed "health," marks the play as an "excellent historie" in which the prospect of disease and the possibility of cure help to drive the plot.

Ceci n'est pas un chien

Of all Shakespeare's characters, only Caliban is more consistently associated with the "brute orders of creation" than Shylock; the Jew is identified repeatedly with dogs and curs in what Boehrer calls a "strain of metaphor...brutally overdetermined" (Boehrer 1999, 161). "Thou called'st me a dog before thou hadst a cause," Shylock says to his tormenters, "But since I am a dog, beware my fangs" (3.3. 6–7). Boehrer emphasizes Shylock's identification first with "slaves and other nonpersons," inverted in the bond of flesh, then as a wolf whose expulsion from England "parallels and prefigures the expulsion of England's Jews" in 1290 (162). He reproduces a still-shocking anti-Semitic image of a German woodcut; in it, two dogs and a Jew hang over a fire in what has been called a "reverse Crucifixion." More recently, Shannon weaves Shakespeare's canine (and lupine) images into a compelling reading about dogs and wolves as "sheep-biters." In Shannon's view, canine hangings indicate "the degree to which 'man's best friend' serves as his likeliest figure for revulsion and violent ejection from human company—paralleling the formal anathemas and excommunications sought in Continental trials."[7] The play, from her perspective, is about the "reach and limits of cosmopolitanism"; a "stranger cur" and sometimes a "wolf," she argues, Shylock stands inside, rather than outside, the "multikinded justiciable cosmos" (241) of Venice. Shylock is like a defendant in animal trials "whose ambivalent status as the stranger within reveals a tension or hypocrisy within a legal system that prides itself on being 'hospitable to diversity'" (246) but that in practice rarely is.[8] In this respect, he is the embodiment and scapegoat of the dog-eat-dog world of Venice's international commerce.

These analyses are enormously helpful in allowing us to see how dogs, wolves, and curs are embedded in a variety of cultural, sociopolitical, and economic discourses. To their readings I would add only this: at stake in *Merchant* is less a particular animal than a Christian agrotheological system. Shylock's shifting status, his fluctuation between dog and wolf, brings him close to assuming the structural position of "vermin" which, as I argued in *Imperfect Creatures*, is not a stable species position but an ontological space readily filled by *any* perceived threat to theological, agricultural, and sociocultural order. Shylock assumes protean figural forms because, like Michel Serres's parasite, he is less a "strange outsider" of a given social order than the necessary precondition for social "order" *as such* (Serres 2007, 9). Christian biopolitics, in other words, *require* vermin, whether they take the form of wolves, dogs, rats, Jews, locusts, or mites. Without a wolf there is no need for a sheep dog; without the threats of disease and predation there is no need for the shepherd; without the wolf and shepherd, there is no need to constitute these herbivores as a flock.

To read the play zoonotically, then, is to begin from an appreciation of real or imaginary contagion as structuring force. Animal trials, segregation

[7] See also Evans (1906) and Dannenfeldt (1982, 542–59).

[8] Shannon, 246. On the legal system, see also Shell (1979, 65–92).

programs, immigration policies—all are built on fears and strategies designed to contain religious, biophysical, and moral infection. Accused across medieval and early modern Europe of poisoning wells or otherwise spreading bubonic plague, Jews were allowed in Venice, but by 1516 had been segregated, forced to live in one of two areas—the *ghetto vecchio* or the *ghetto nuovo*—in the *Cannaregio sestiere*, which also housed the municipal slaughterhouses. The connection between Jews and dogs that we see in *Merchant* was both common and steeped in the logics of quarantines, culling, and vermin eradication.

Dogs were subject to containment strategies all over Europe, policies justified implicitly and explicitly by dogs' wandering and their indiscriminate feeding practices. A popular plague book reprinted in 1603 advocates that people "keep their houses, street, yards, and sinks, and ditches sweet and clean from all standing puddles, dunghills, and corrupt moistures" in order to prevent outbreaks and that dogs not be allowed to run in the house, since these "will be most apt cattle ... to carry the infection" from standing water and waste (Mullett 1937, 325–27). In 1636, London exterminated 3720 dogs, feral animals that, according to Mark Jenner, were perceived as "visible sources of disorder, out of control and unsanitary" (Jenner 1997, 50). As street scavengers, feral dogs fed on carrion, including fallen or carelessly buried infected cattle, which meant that during nonhuman or epizootic outbreaks, they were similarly forced into regimes of containment, hygiene, and control (Cole 2016, 136–138; Spinage 2003, 177, 167). In 1556 Prussia forbade "the loading of dogs with cattle skins" in an attempt to stop the spread of a raging cattle disease, and a 1604 ordinance in Lyon issued during a cattle outbreak ordered the slaughter of stray dogs (Spinage, 98). The carrion-eating habits of dogs also helped reinforce the logic of pit burials. Mascall's *First booke of cattell* recommends flaying or skinning an infected animal, burying it in a "deepe pitte," covering it within enough earth to disguise the smell from carrion-eating dogs, and carrying the skin straight to the tanner rather than home (67). Mascall warns that many people believe the more prudent course is to bury the carcass whole. In his description, the livestock, dog, butcher, and tanner may be mutually and fatally infected, caught up in a multispecies cycle of contagion, a perception that grew stronger as outbreaks multiplied in the eighteenth century.[9] A 1743 Metz ordinance

[9] During a nineteenth-century outbreak, Austria paid special attention to its "frontiers": "Any wandering, masterless dogs near the frontiers were to be shot" (Spinage 265). Although

ordered that dogs on infected farms either be tied up or shot (Spinage 117). In 1745, the King of Denmark and Norway ordered not only "the shooting of all cats and dogs on infected farms and confinement of pigs, sheep, and geese," but commanded that all animals and people be washed in vinegar water and quarantined for 14 days (Spinage 247).

Admittedly, there is nothing at first glance about infection or disease in Gratiano's much-cited, anti-Semitic description of Shylock: "Thy currish spirit," he vituperates,

> Govern'd a wolf, who hang'd for human slaughter,
> Even from the gallows did his fell soul fleet,
> And whilst thou layest in thy unhallowed dam,
> Infus'd itself in thee; for thy desires
> Are wolvish, bloody, starv'd, and ravenous. (4.1. 128–38)

The last word, "ravenous," describes a predatory hunger and serves as a synonym for a "starv'd" and rapacious animal, literal or figurative. Significantly, however, a now obsolete meaning of "ravenous" is "rabid." As Topsell writes, "A ravening Wolfe by his biting bringeth the same danger, as a ravenous Dogge" (584). This definition is critical because rabid dogs and wolves presented early modern readers with the only unequivocal example of zoonotic disease—the clearest evidence of how humans and animals are vulnerable to the same neurological maladies.[10] Indeed, rabies often was described as an "an ungovernable fury," and, before 1700, no clear distinction existed between the psychological state of being furious and the medical diagnosis of rabid, bodily infection. In fact, the term "rabies" (from the Latin *rabere*, "be mad, rave") was at first applied primarily to humans and only secondarily to dogs, although the relationship was always close. When Edgar in *King Lear* assumes the character of Poor Tom, a "Bedlam beggar," he "shift[s]/ Into a madman's rags, t'assume a semblance/ That very dogs disdained" (5.3. 181–183). In his performance as Tom o' Bedlam, he imagines himself embedded in a pack of dogs, behaving like them even threatening to outdo them: "Avaunt, you curs!"

these last and especially draconian regulations were intended to protect against what by then had been identified as rinderpest, premodern, early modern, and modern European practice share a history of canine regulation in relation to zoonotic and epizootic disease.

[10] Historical accounts of rabies include Blaisdell (1991, 22–23); and Pemberton and Warboys (2007).

Be thy mouth or black or white,
Tooth that poisons if it bite;
Mastiff, greyhound, mongrel grim,
Hound or spaniel, brach, or him,
Bobtail tyke or trundle-tail—
Tom will make them weep and wail. (3.6. 20–26)

To disguise his identity, Tom assumes, in the words of an eighteenth-century treatise on rabies, the hallmarks of the most "dreadful disease incident to human nature" (Layard 1762, 4). When Shylock warns, "But since I am a dog, beware my fangs," he does something similar: he both evokes and protests his having been marked as a ravenous—that is, *contagious*—animal who must be contained or exterminated.

In the context of contemporary husbandry manuals, we can see how Shylock's behavior seems to fit the criteria that characterize a rabid man: "For of him that is bitten," writes Mascall, "the venome goeth from the bitten place to the heart, & from thence to the head" (196). Infection leads directly from contagion to madness: "it is also daungerous to touch those bodies infected, because the vaporation and vehemencie of the venome, and they will corrupt all things neere unto them" (196). Rabies follows this logic of epidemiological and moral contagion. In *Merchant*, Shylock's implied status as potentially rabid is conveyed by a set of related images about indiscriminate feeding practices, widely imagined, in the sixteenth century, as a likely source of both rabies and bubonic plague. When Shylock tells Jessica that he goes to supper with Antonio "in hate to feed upon/ The prodigal Christian" (2.5. 11–12), he introduces a pattern of feeding that aligns him with wolves *and* dogs, and runs counter to God's commandments to the Jews: "And you shall be holy men unto me: neither shall ye eat any flesh that is torn of beasts in the field; ye shall cast it to the dogs" (Exodus 22: 31). In Old and New Testament passages, both dogs and wolves appear as stand-ins for treacherous humans, such as in Phillipians 3:2: "Watch out for those dogs, those evildoers, those mutilators of the flesh." When Salarino, in disbelief, asks why he would take Antonio's pound of flesh—"what's that good for?"—Shylock doubles down on the entwined rhetorics of scavenging and outrage: "If it will feed nothing else, it will feed my revenge" (3.1.52). As the play moves toward the trial scene, differences between the language of Shylock's fury and his rapacious feeding practices seem to disappear. At the trial, he justifies as his "humor" his insistence on preferring a "weight of carrion flesh" over three thousand ducats, embracing the image of himself as a rabid animal, "governed by fury," unleashing his desire to mutilate Antonio's body: "So can I give no reason, nor I will not/ More than a lodged hate and certain loathing/ I bear Antonio, that I follow thus/ A losing suit against him" (4.1.35–8). At this point he is "ravenous" in every contemporary sense of the word—covetous, furious, diseased, mad—and therefore in need of containment and care: *A righteous man hath regard for the life of his beast.* But this regard is overdetermined by the antisemitism and moral certainty of the Christian community.

Canine containment, like lupine eradication before it, was designed to protect both a fearful and susceptible human population and a lucrative yet vulnerable meat market. *The Merchant of Venice*, I have argued, participates in this multilayered discourse on several levels—theological, economic, and agricultural: care for domestic animals, moral and theological imperatives to guard and sustain the flock or herd, and best practices to maximize profits from meat, hides, and fleece. When Shylock warns "But since I am a dog, beware my fangs" (3.3.5), he both evokes and protests against his having been marked as a contagious animal that has to be contained and threatened with extermination. But his poignant appeals to species-level identification among all humans cut both ways. While some of his questions point to a common sensibility as well as biophysical identity—"Hath not a Jew eyes? Hath not a Jew hands, organs, dimensions, senses, affections, passions?" (3.1.52–3)—others remind his audience about the anti-Semitic stereotypes associated with an early modern zoonotic imaginary. Are we not "fed with the same food," he asks, "hurt with same weapons, subject to the same diseases, healed by the same means, warmed and cooled by the same winter and summer as a Christian is?. . . If you prick us, do we not bleed? If you poison us, do we not die?" (3.1.52–4). This appeal to shared biophysical experiences can be and has been read as Shylock pleading for an acknowledgment of his humanity. But his comparisons between Jew and Christian also raise the specter that, in the words of Francis Bacon, "Man is of kinne to the Beast by his Body" (1663, 91). Shylock is outwitted by Portia for his rigid adherence to what he assumes is the letter of the law, and is caught in his own assumption that the laws of Venice cannot be turned against him as the holder of the bond. Forced to relinquish his religion and his riches, he must be neutralized as a threat, as a source of moral, theological, economic, and cultural contagion. In the context of multispecies contagion, then, Shylock's poignant call for a common humanity might be regarded more accurately as a guarantee of its limits: a shared susceptibility to the coercive aspects of pastoral power.

Reading Zoonotically

We share with early moderns the experience of living in a cosmopolitan world rife with zoonotic and epizootic diseases, with what they called "great mortalities of both man and beast." We also share the experience—I have argued—of a vulnerable trade in animal flesh, one threatened at every moment by contagions and afflictions requiring constant vigilance. I don't want to end this chapter, though, with the impression that reading zoonotically means placing literature, like a stencil, over a disease-ridden "background"; instead, I want to emphasize that husbandry manuals, sermons, plays, art, and medical treatises, with animal trials and other legal practices, constitute a complex set of discourses that serve as the impetus and interpretive space for a medical posthumanities. Zoonotic reading attends to specific diseases and the practices, including strategic killing, intended to confront them. Sometimes these diseases are named (Ajax's "scab") and sometimes not (Antonio's "taint").

While writing this chapter, I puzzled over a 1655 etching by Karel Dujardin (1622–1678), an artist born in Amsterdam, who trained in Rome, and died in Venice. Dujardin is mostly known as landscape painter who, like many of his contemporaries, produces rural genre scenes: "Woman Milking a Cow," "Farm Animals in the Shade of a Tree," "Three Pigs in a Hedge." Consider, however, the engraving called "Sheep With Flies," "Recumbent Sheep With Flies," or (in the version on Artstor, from the Metropolitan Museum of Art) "Partially shorn sheep lying in the grass with insects hovering around its head" (Fig. 3.1).

The shepherd is a vague figure in the landscape (right) looking toward his feeding flock on the hill to the viewer's left. Isolated from the flock, the sheep in the foreground offers an epidemiological puzzle.

Artstor's (possible AI-generated) description of this etching seems to me inaccurate. The sheep's wool is not "partially shorn," as in the title, but torn off or massively shedding. Markham's description of "unsoundess" in sheep includes "eyes heavy and darke," and the observation that "its wooll" when pulled will easily part from the sheep's body (71). Although the cloud of flies around the animal's head could indicate fly-strike, an infestation associated with damp or dirty fleece, the sheep is likely afflicted

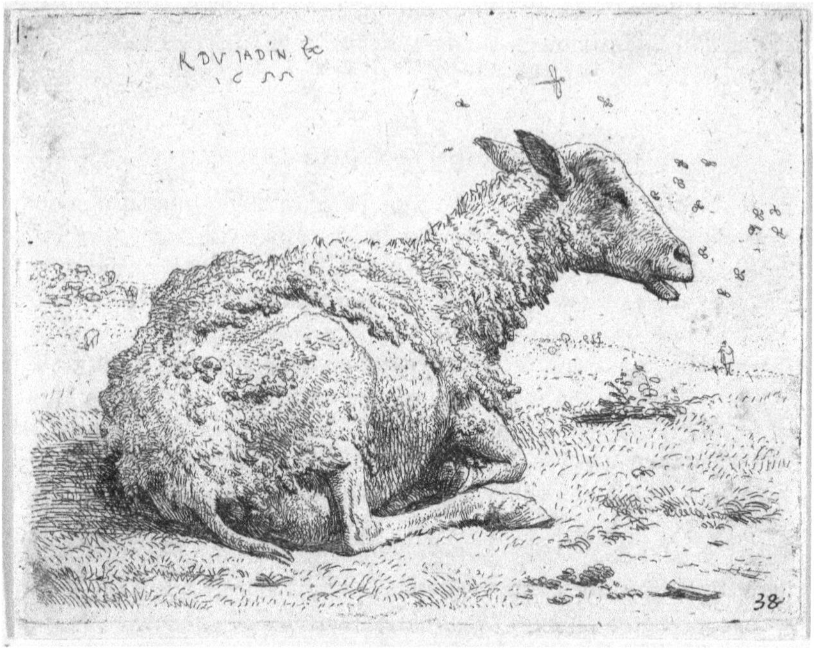

Fig. 3.1 *Partially shorn sheep lying in the grass with insects hovering around its head.* Karel Dujardin, 1655. Metropolitan Museum of Art

with scab, the pathological darling of pastoral biopolitics. Clinical signs of the disease include itching that leads the sheep to biting at its flanks, or "nibbling," loss of wool, and secondary skin infections—"known," as Markham says, "by a white filthy scurfe sticking vpon their skins" (71). The purulent or oozing wounds, in turn, attract flies, prominently depicted here. Moreover, among contemporary clinical symptoms of scab is a desire for solitude, a point emphasized by Topsell, Markham, and other writers on animal husbandry. Understanding the prevalence and significance of animal diseases, in short, changes how we read this etching.

The significance of this estranged scabbed sheep is, of course, debatable. It seems to present pictorially a contagion scene from Virgil's Georgics (here, in Dryden's translation):

> But where thou seest a single Sheep remain
> In shades aloof, or couch'd upon the Plain;
> Or listlessly to crop the tender Grass;

> Or late to lag behind, with truant pace;
> Revenge the Crime; and take the Traytor's head,
> E're in the faultless Flock the dire Contagion spread. (Dryden 1697, ll. 705–710)

Perhaps, then, Dujardin illustrates the familiar proverb: "one scabbed sheep will ruin the whole flock," which—especially during the politically volatile seventeenth century—would be resurrected as a running theme of sermons against "Christ-mocking."[11] Perhaps it is a religious allegory along the lines of Wood, a reminder—via Psalm 23—of our collective vulnerability to and necessity for a watchful shepherd. In either case, though, the very possibility of figural meaning depends on the viewer's ability to *see* animal diseases and recognize their potential zoonotic implications. If we retreat to the rhetoric of aesthetic categories, we end up rendering pastoral biopolitics tangential. "The *pointe* of Karel the engraver," according to an anonymous nineteenth-century art critic, "is always picturesque"; he points to the "differences and contrasts of reality, the dirty wool of the sheep, the knotted and entangled fleeces" (1854, 260). According to these categories, Karel's scene is picturesque in contrast to the beautiful; in William Gilpin's sense, picturesque objects "please the eye" not from some quality in their "natural state" but "from some quality, capable of being illustrated by painting" (Gilpin 1792, 3). Insofar as aesthetic categories occlude disease, or reframe a scabbed sheep as a "Partially shorn sheep lying in the grass with insects hovering around its head," they cover over, or prepare for aesthetic consumption, the realities of the trade in flesh, fleece, and hides.

Zoonotic reading allows us to comprehend the fleshiness of the animal trade. This chapter has treated part of that trade as an arm of pastoral biopolitics and its assemblages, including the medical relationship between a shepherd and his vulnerable flock, both susceptible to cross-species contagion. In all its forms, though, zoonotic reading requires us to reject the idea that contagion, infection, and other signs of transcorporeality are negative and opposed to identity, essence, and coherence. To borrow the words of Roberto Marchesini, "it is not possible to find assonance with the biosphere while remaining attached to a paradigm that denies the elementary logic of life" (Marchesini 2021, 57). Zoonotic reading treats viruses, bacteria, and insects as actors; it acknowledges that we—humans and

[11] On scabbed seep and false doctrine see, for example, Clarke (1646, 15).

animals—are alike in "eyes" and "organs," that we are often "subject," in Shylock's words, to the same diseases. In this sense, zoonotic reading takes place through and across the rhetorics of disciplinary knowledge. Although early modern literature is open to this reality and its correspondent hermeneutics, zoonotic reading is subject to counterforces, many of those forged during the Enlightenment. The next chapters attend to the absences, silences, displacements, erasures, and blindnesses—intentional or otherwise—that have ensured the "humanness" of the medical humanities, the "literariness" of literature, and the "thingness" of histories on, say, the commercial wool trade, in which the protective covering of living animals is treated simply as another commodity fetish.

References

Appuhn, Karl. 2010. Ecologies of Beef: Eighteenth-Century Epizootics and the Environmental History of Early Modern Europe. *Environmental History* 15 (2): 268–287.

Bacon, Francis. 1663. Of Atheism. In *The essays, or, Counsels, civil and moral, of Sir Francis Bacon*. London: J. Redmayne for Thomas Palmer.

Blaisdell, John. 1991. Rabies in Shakespeare's England. *Historia Medicinae Veterinariae* 16:1–48.

Blanchard, Ian. 1986. The Continental European Cattle Trades. *The Economic History Review* 39:427–460.

Boehrer, Bruce. 1999. Shylock and the Rise of the Household Pet: Thinking Social Exclusion in *The Merchant of Venice*. *Shakespeare Quarterly* 50:152–170.

Boehrer, Bruce. 2010. *Animal Characters: Nonhuman Beings in the Early Modern World*. Philadelphia: University of Pennsylvania Press.

Clarke, John. 1646. *Leaven, corrupting the Childrens Bread; or Christs caveat to beware of sectaries and their dangerous doctrines*. London: Printed by John Macock for Luke Fawne.

Cole, Lucinda. 2016. *Imperfect Creatures: Vermin, Literature, and the Science of Life 1600–1740*. Ann Arbor: University of Michigan Press.

Cole, Lucinda. 2023. Out of Africa: Locust Infestation, Universal History, and the Early Modern Theological Imaginary. In *Lesser Creatures of the Renaissance*, ed. Keith Botelho and Joseph Campana, vol. 2, 62–82. State College: Pennsylvania State University Press.

Collins, Samuel. 1685. *A systeme of anatomy, treating of the body of man, beasts, birds, fish, insects, and plants*. London: Thomas Newcomb.

Dannenfeldt, Karl H. 1982. The Control of Vertebrate Pests in Renaissance Agriculture. *Agricultural History* 56:542–559.

Dryden, John. 1697. *The Works of Virgil, containing his Pastorals, Georgics, and Aeneis*. London: Jacob Tonson.
Duncan-Jones, Katherine. 2004. Did the Boy Shakespeare Kill Calves? *Review of English Studies* (new series) 55:183–195.
Evans, E. P. 1906. *The Criminal Prosecution and Capital Punishment of Animals*. London: Heinemann.
Foucault, Michel. 2007. *Security, Territory, Population: Lectures at the College de France, 177–1978*. Translated by Graham Burchell. New York: Picador.
Galloway, James A., and Margaret Murphy. 1991. Feeding the City: Medieval London and its Agrarian Hinterland. *The London Journal* 16 (1): 3–14.
Gilpin, William. 1792. *Three essays: On picturesque beauty; on picturesque travel; and on sketching landscape*. London: R. Blamire.
Giromani, Virgilio. 2004. The Lido as Venice's Refuse Tip: Dalmatian Sheep and the 1819 Elephant. *Historia Medicinae Veterinariae* 29 (1): 3–12.
Greenblatt, Stephen, Walter Cohen, Jean E. Howard, and Katherine Eisaman Maus. 1997. *The Norton Shakespeare: Based on the Oxford Edition*. New York: Norton.
Harris, Jonathan Gil. 1998. 'The Enterprise is Sick': Pathologies of Value and Transnationality in *Troilus and Cressida*. *Renaissance Drama* 29:3–37.
Hirota, Atsuhiko. 2017. Venetian Jasons, Parti-coloured Lambs, and a Tainted Wether: Ovine Tropes and the Golden Fleece in *The Merchant of Venice*. In *Interweaving Myths in Shakespeare and His Contemporaries*, ed. Janice Valls-Russell, Agnes Lafont, and Charlotte Coffin. Manchester: Manchester University Press.
Illustrated Magazine of Art. 1854. 3, 16: 260.
Jenner, Mark. 1997. The Great Dog Massacre. In *Fear in Early Modern Society*, ed. William G. Naphy and Penny Roberts, 44–61. New York: St. Martin's Press.
Layard, Daniel Peter. 1762. *An Essay on the Bite of a Mad Dog*. London: John Rivington and Thomas Payne.
Marchesini, Roberto. 2021. *The Virus Paradigm: A Planetary Ecology of Mind*. Translated by Sarah De Sanctis. Cambridge: Cambridge University Press.
Markham, Gervase. 1614. *Cheape and good husbandry for the well-ordering of all beasts and fowls, and for the general cure of their diseases*. London: T.S. for Roger Jackson.
Mascall, Leonard. 1587. *The first booke of cattell*. London: Iohn Wolfe.
McGinnes, Ian F. 2020. Cow Cross Lane and Curriers Row: Animal Networks in Early Modern England. In *Routledge Handbook of Shakespeare and Animals*, ed. Karen Raber and Holly Dugan. New York: Routledge.
Mullett, Charles. 1937. Some Neglected Aspects of Plague Medicine in Sixteenth-Century England. *Scientific Monthly* 44 (4): 325–337.
Pemberton, Neil, and Michael Warboys. 2007. *Dogs, Diseases and Culture, 1830–2000*. Basingstoke: Palgrave Macmillan.

Raber, Karen. 2013. *Animal Bodies, Renaissance Culture*. Philadelphia: University of Pennsylvania Press.
Ray, John. 1678. *A Collection of English Proverbs*. 2nd ed. Cambridge: Printed by John Hayes for W. Morden.
Schoenbaum, Samuel. 1975. *William Shakespeare: A Documentary Life*. Oxford: Clarendon.
Serres, Michel. 2007. *The Parasite*. Translated by Lawrence Scher. Minneapolis: University of Minnesota Press.
Shannon, Laurie. 2013. *The Accommodated Animal: Cosmopolity in Shakespearean Locales*. Chicago: University of Chicago Press.
Shell, Marc. 1979. The Wether and the Ewe: Verbal Usury in *The Merchant of Venice*. *Kenyon Review* (new series) 1 (4): 65–92.
Shrewsbury, J. F. D. 1950. The Plague of Athens. *Bulletin of the History of Medicine* 24:1–25.
Spinage, Clive. 2003. *Cattle Plague: A History*. Amsterdam: Kluwer Academic/ Plenum Publishers.
Topsell, Edward. 1658. *The history of four-footed beasts and serpents . . . whereunto is now added, The theater of insects, or, Lesser living creatures* . . . by T. Muffet. London: E. Cotes for G. Sawbridge.
Webster, Noah. 1799. *A brief history of epidemic and pestilential diseases*. Hartford, CT: Hudson and Goodwin.
Wilkinson, Lise. 1980. Veterinary Cross-currents in the History of Ideas on Infectious Disease. *Journal of the Royal Society of Medicine* 73:818–827.
Wilkinson, Lise. 1992. *Animals and Epidemics: An Introduction to the History of Comparative Medicine*. Cambridge: Cambridge University Press.
Woode, James. 1680. *Sheperdy Spiritualiz'd or, The Improvement of a Shepherd's Life to Soul-Advantage*. London: J. R. for Thomas Parkhurst.
Yates, Julian. 2017. *Of Sheep, Oranges, and Yeasts: A Multispecies Impression*. Minneapolis: University of Minnesota Press.

CHAPTER 4

Journals of the Plague Years: Flesh Markets and Easterly Winds

Abstract Between 1711 and 1769, more than 200 million cattle in Western Europe succumbed to a variety of diseases. A growing international cattle trade ensured that pandemics became transnational epidemiological and ecological crises. Chapter 4 begins by examining depictions of cattle plague in treatises about the 1720 bubonic plague at Marseilles, which was preceded by widespread outbreaks of cattle disease; these texts include Richard Bradley's *The plague at Marseilles considered, with remarks upon the plague in general, shewing its causes and nature of infection* (1721) and Nathaniel Hodges's updated *Loimologia, or an historical account of the plague in London in 1665* (1720). All consider at length possible relationships between mass cattle die-offs and human disease. The works of Daniel Defoe, by contrast, exhibit a deep anxiety about meat and meat markets, especially meat imported from the Eurasian steppes. With their huge herds of horses, sheep, cattle, and camels, the steppes began in the seventeenth century to occupy the geopathological position formerly represented by a presumably noxious Nile Delta. I examine reports of what was probably anthrax in travel writers in the seventeenth and eighteenth centuries, linking those to Defoe's derogatory comments about "Tartars" in his plague writings, and to Crusoe's dramatic attack on the Tartar "idol" Cham Chi-Thaungu in *Farther Adventures of Robinson Crusoe* (1719).

L. Cole, *The Fifth Plague*, Palgrave Studies in Animals and Literature, https://doi.org/10.1007/978-3-031-92793-5_4

Can anything help Nature against the God of Nature?
—William Kemp, *A brief treatise of the nature, causes, signes, preservation from, and cure of the pestilence* (1665)

Livestock disease, as we saw in *The Merchant of Venice*, is deeply entangled with ethical, economic, and political reality. Writing as Issac Bickerstaff, Defoe offers as one of twelve "prophesies" for 1711 that, because "*Italy* and *Germany*" and other "populous nations on that side" have "felt the fury of the Contagion," Britain should prepare itself for a similar "Plague." Echoing Exodus 9:3, Bickerstaff declares that "a great Rot falls among the Court-Sheep" in this nation, and "a Murrain upon the Stallions of this *Sodomitish* City. The Infection spares none" (Defoe 1711, 10). Defoe's extended metaphor acquires much of its force from an ongoing epizootic, with livestock diseases circulating and recirculating throughout Europe. His figurative warning about a furious multispecies contagion invading Britain, although directed at bestial politicians, captures a critical truth for his eighteenth-century readers. Animal plagues, rot and murrain among them, are never simply about the welfare of animals, but about the knock-on effects that threaten livestock prices, food supplies, local and national economic stability, and domestic and foreign trade. Moreover, during Defoe's lifetime treatise after treatise took up the key question of zoonotic transmission: did cattle plagues lead to outbreaks of human disease, particularly bubonic plague?

During the eighteenth century, England suffered three cattle pandemics, usually described as occurring from 1709 to 1720; 1742 to 1760; and 1768 to 1786. In 1711—the year of Defoe's "vision"—rinderpest found its way from Tartary, through Hungary, to herds at Padua, presumably (and perhaps apocryphally) from one stray Dalmatian ox; by October the disease had enveloped the "length and breadth of the Venetia" and was "raging with undiminished force" (Wilkinson 1984, 131; Wilkinson 1992, 35–64). Seeking to stamp out, or at least contain, the outbreak, the Venetian Senate turned to the medical faculty at the University of Padua for help. Its principal Professor of Medicine, Bernandino Ramazzini (1633–1714), wrote a broadside chastising medical men who, he says, wrongly thought it beneath their dignity to attend to cattle; for the sake of public health, he insists, all sick cattle should be culled, killed, and buried (Franco 2020, 321–325). Two years later, with disease still raging, another Italian physician, Giovanni Maria Lancisi (1654–1720), took up the public health project. On Lancisi's recommendation, Pope Clement XI wrote and delivered a series of edicts prohibiting the trade in meat, hides, and fat of infected animals. Penalties for disobeying the Pope's proscriptions included death by hanging, but, despite such draconian measures, the Venetian plague spread to the continent and, via Holland, to England. Thomas Bates, Surgeon to King George, had been stationed in Sicily during the initial Italian outbreak (Spinage 2003, 112). Placed in charge of containing the contagion in England, Bates more or less replicated Italy's policies (Broad 1983, 40). Between 1711 and 1714 over a million and a half cattle died, either from the disease or from slaughter policies intended to mitigate the transmission of the disease (Mullet 1946, 144–165; Spinage 104–114). The first plague in England ended fairly quickly, writes Clive Spinage, for several reasons: because of mandated cattle culls; because "no one would buy a cow in the country for fear of the disease"; and because, in the towns, markets were inspected daily "and meat which appeared suspicious condemned" (112). To borrow Defoe's words, the "Infection" spared none.

In this chapter, I focus on outbreaks from 1709 to 1720 and the plague treatises they engendered, before moving on to consider the later eighteenth-century cattle plagues in Chap. 5. These early-century outbreaks were associated with, if not bookended by, two eruptions of bubonic plague, the first in London (1665) and the second in Marseilles (1720). Between May of 1720 and March of 1721, bubonic plague claimed 40,000 victims in Marseilles and its environs (Mullet 1936, 484). Richard Bradley reports that one physician arrived to a nightmare scene in the city, finding its people "without Bread, without Wine, without Meat, without Medicines" (1721, viii) and the streets reeking of dead human *and* animal bodies. Contemporary accounts indicate that 4000 people may have died in a single day. Cindy Ermus identifies the plague in Marseilles as Europe's first "modern" disaster, in that it provoked widespread coordination of disaster management, what she terms "disaster centralism" (Ermus 2022, 5–6). France eventually built a plague wall to separate the city from the rest of Provence. Because the plague at Marseilles was preceded by an epizootic event, it dramatically shook a widespread but unstable belief that cattle plagues were not fatal to humans and human plagues not fatal to cattle.

Given that epidemiological relationships between epizootic outbreaks and bubonic plague were imperfectly understood, physicians, officials, and citizens were forced to deal with at least three overlapping sets of concerns and strategies: (1) whether quarantine strategies applied to animals during cattle disease outbreaks could or should be applied to humans, or vice versa; (2) whether diseased animal products or even venomous insects could transmit both human and animal plague; and (3) whether humans and livestock could fall victim to the same illnesses. The last question proved to be especially tricky. While it would eventually become clear that what the British called "cattle plague" and what we, after the Germans, call "rinderpest" could *not* be spread to humans, anthrax could; as for foot and mouth disease—it's complicated. In language that often swept all mass mortalities under the rubric of "pestilence," Richard Mead (*A short discourse concerning pestilential contagion*, 1720), John Quincy (*Essay on the different causes of pestilential diseases, and how they became contagious*, 1721), and Richard Bradley (*The plague at Marseilles considered*, 1721) wrote treatises that help to define the contours of this multispecies epidemiological and socioeconomic crisis.

I invoke Daniel Defoe's *Journal of the Plague Year* (1722a) in the title of this chapter, though, because I also want to explore how this novel—a touchstone for the medical humanities as a discipline—redirects the debates about cross-species contagion away from cattle plague proper to focus on London's socioeconomic vulnerabilities during the 1665 plague. The first section of this chapter, then, discusses some of the medical debates about zoonotic transmission, beginning with Nathaniel Hodges's *Loimologia*, written during the 1665 visitation and republished with Quincy's *An Essay on the different causes of pestilential diseases, and how they became contagious* in 1720. Competing views about the direct transmission of disease across species, I suggest, are often subsumed within larger fears about humans catching the plague from infected animal skins, tainted meat, or other tradable goods. Next, I turn to Defoe in sections devoted, first, to *Journal of the Plague Year* and, second, to *Farther Adventures of Robinson Crusoe* (1719). Unlike Mead, Quincy, and Bradley, conversant with the contours of an increasingly international livestock trade, Defoe tends to condense theoretical concerns about cross-species infection into a single industry problem: corrupted meat. His anxiety about meat and meat markets—also evident in Richard Blackmore's *A discourse upon the plague, with a preparatory account of malignant fevers* (1721)—runs through Defoe's *Journal of the Plague Year*, *Due Preparations for the Plague* (1722b), and even *Farther Adventures of Robinson Crusoe*. In this 1719 novel, Crusoe's caravan journey from China, across Siberia and Russia, to Archangel on the Baltic coast reveals Defoe's fears about the Eurasian steppes as a source of disease, corruption, and idolatry. In the seventeenth century, huge herds of horses, sheep, cattle, and camels, stretching across the grasslands from eastern Europe to Manchuria, had begun to occupy the geo-pathological position earlier represented by a presumably noxious Nile Delta; by the early eighteenth century, fears about the threat of "steppe diseases" either replace—or coexist with—the plagues of Egypt in the popular imagination. While these fears were caught up in the complicated politics of Catholic and Protestant confrontations with Islamic cultures, concerns about the consequences of the international trade in cattle from Asia to Europe persisted for two centuries.[1]

The first reference to "step" as a geographical location in the OED cites Samuel Collins's *The present state of Russia* (1671), where it connotes a vast "wilderness." Collins describes the nomadic inhabitants of the steppes "as quick-sighted as any people in the world, and will descry upon the Step or Wilderness (where a man hath nothing to hinder his prospect thirty or forty miles round) I say, they will descry a single man, when a Russ cannot see a whole troop of Tartars" (88). The steppes—without property markers, trees, or mountains—and its peoples function as the agricultural and spiritual others of "civilized" Europe. Eighteenth-century travel narratives about the Czar's empire intensified such perceptions. In different ways, Evert Isbrant Ides, *Three years travels from Moscow over-land to China* (translated into English in 1706); John Bell, *Travels from St. Petersburg in Russia to diverse Parts of Asia* (1720, but not published until 1763); the English translations and digests of the German naturalist, Peter Simon Pallas (incorporated into the histories of Russia by William Coxe and William Tooke) and John Trusler's multi-volumed compendium, *The habitable world described* (1788–97) all cast the steppes as the noxious source of disease-carrying livestock.[2] Such travel narratives, read alongside

[1] On the complex border politics of these regions in the eighteenth century, see Garcia (2010, 1–25).

[2] Pallas lived in Russia for most of his adult life and made two extended scientific journeys in 1768–74 and 1793–4 to the Ural Mountains and parts of southern and western Siberia. The first full English translation of the latter journey was by Fancis Blagdon as *Travels through the Southern Provinces of the Russian Empire, in the years 1793 and 1794* (1802). Accounts of the earlier expedition were incorporated by both William Coxe, *Account of the Russian Discoveries between Asia and America* (1780), and William Tooke, *View of the Russian Empire during the Reign of Catharine the Second, and to the Close of the Present Century* (1799). Because both Coxe and Tooke drew on other travel accounts as well as their own experiences in Russia, the narrative "I" in their texts is sometimes syncretic and not necessarily a single account. Trusler's text incorporates parts of their translations and separate contributions to the *Philosophical Transactions*. Because my concern in this chapter is with observations of human and cattle disease and wider perceptions of so-called steppe disease, I quote from Trusler's popular *Habitable World*.

European plague journals, reveal how Western Europe's increasing dependence on outsourced grazing operations made references to pestilential "*East*-winds" or "*Easterly* winds" as a kind of shorthand for cattle plague. Even though Defoe marginalizes direct references to cattle disease, his works were written during a period of intense concern with the health of England's herds, and his biases about the steppes and its nomadic peoples are of a piece with these travel narratives; they help suture perceptions of "filthy Tartars," eastern grazing operations, and corrupted meat to matters of public health. Much later, such attitudes helped to justify and set into motion colonial sanitary measures deployed across Eurasia, measures intended to safeguard Christian Europe against peoples and their livestock regarded as endemically infectious.

Debates About Zoonotic Contagion

Because bubonic plague often followed outbreaks of livestock disease, cattle plagues fueled often widespread fears of cross-species infection. Nathaniel Hodges's *Loimologia, or an historical account of the plague in London in 1665* offers several anecdotes that center on sick animals and infected people. Hodges cites several instances of apparent cross-species contagion. A "certain Leech" or cow-doctor opens a horse that had died "with a great many others of some common Distemper"; the "Master" of the horse, seeing some "pestilential Tokens" on the horse's "Inwards" died, followed by his entire family (60). A second tale reports that during the "late *Plague*" in London a citizen who traveled into the country on horseback found "his Horse of a sudden to tire and fall down"; after opening the animal's mouth, "upon Receipt of the Horse's Breath upon him," he "immediately grew sick, and died in two Days Time" (61). Such cases, Hodges argues, prove a possible human susceptibility to livestock disease, which he explains in the convoluted language of humoral theory: "Constitutions and malignant Steams, which, by agitating the Mass of Humours, may excite putrid and irregular Orgasms, wherein the Juices and Animal Fluids, according to the Quantity and Prevalency of the Distemperature, and the Variety of the infused Taint, with the Diversity of Putrefaction, goes into Corruption" (61). But such reports do not demonstrate unequivocally that murrain can infect humans: "the Conjecture that a Sickness amongst Cattle is transferable to the humane Species," he asserts, "hath not yet appeared on any good Foundation" (60). Although Hodges "cannot be induced to believe" that "Pestilence amongst Cattle from a private Cause" can ever "obtain any Dominion over Mankind," he hedges his bet by holding open the possibility that plagues may be similar enough, under the right circumstances, to afflict humans and nonhuman animals alike: "a Plague amongst Cattle, from some common Cause," he writes, "as a Corruption of the aerial Nitre, and which differs from a Plague amongst Men but in Degree, may also be transmitted to the humane Species" (60). At stake in his distinction between "private" and "common" causes is "the epidemic constitution" of miasma theory; because humans and nonhumans share "animal spirits," should they be exposed to the same environmental conditions, they could be similarly afflicted.[3] In short, Hodges rejects popular stories about direct transmission of cattle disease to humans, but agrees that humans and cattle can both become victims of a common disease vector, like bad air, even if they respond differently. Miasma theory, in this respect, becomes a way for seventeenth- and eighteenth-century writers to think about environmental factors in disease transmission and mitigation, including air pollution (Cavert 2016, 32–41).

In the first decades of the eighteenth century, called upon to help mitigate enzootic outbreaks around Italy, the Italian physicians Ramazzini and Lancisi also took seriously the question of whether cattle plagues could cross species boundaries. While acknowledging similarities between cattle plague and human smallpox, Ramazzini, in contrast to many of his predecessors, argues that the former affected only cattle. Yet, like his sixteenth-century predecessor, Leonard Mascall, he nevertheless insists that humans could carry the disease.[4] Lancisi similarly describes cattle plague as a kind of "poison" passing from beast to beast but one that could be transmitted by "other animals, birds, and men" (Mullet 1946, 145, n 4). Embedded in both accounts are concerns about zoonosis or, more precisely, reverse zoonosis, the transmittal of disease from humans to animals.

During the outbreak of bubonic plague in Marseilles such assumptions were put to experimental verification. The *Philosophical Transactions of the Royal Society* reports that a French physician, Dr. Deidier, had extracted bile from the gall bladders of people who had succumbed to the plague; he then "poured" the bile "into a Wound made on Purpose in different Dogs," all of whom died in three or four days, "with the essential Marks of the true Plague"—"Buboes, Carbuncles, and gangrenous Inflammation

[3] On aerial niter, see Debus (1964: 43–61).

[4] Mullet (1946, 145). See Williamson (1958) on Deidier.

in the Viscera, in the same manner as the human Carcasses from which the Bile was taken" (Eames and Martin 1734, 2: 595). This article also describes a dog who lived in the Marseilles hospital, following the doctors and licking up blood after surgeries, who was subjected to a similar trial. The unnamed dog had always been "well, gay, brisk, full of Play, and familiar with all Comers," but after the physicians injected him with a dram of the same "pestiferous bile," he too died the fourth day, with a bubo, then two carbuncles. Finally, Deidier and his colleagues transferred bile from a dog dead of the plague into an apparently healthy dog, with similarly fatal results (2: 595–96). Although bubonic plague is rare in dogs, as we now know, it can be transmitted either through an intermediary disease vector or directly, as these grim experiments demonstrate. John Mullet points to such tests as refuting the contemporary belief that early plague science was "scarcely more than magic" (Mullet 1936, 514). I would add that experiments designed to refute or verify cross-species contagion attest to an awareness that human and animal health in a cattle-grain economy are deeply entangled, so entangled that physicians during this period rarely address bubonic plague or cattle plague without at least considering contemporary evidence of zoonotic transmission.

The threat of Marseille's plague spreading to England intensified pressure on English medical writers to clarify the relationship between livestock and human diseases. Thomas Bates, writing about a 1714 contagious disease in cows had acknowledged that the "Nature of Contagious Diseases are but little understood" but posited cattle-to-human infection as a rarity. "The Providence of God has so disposed of the matter of Animal Bodies," he writes, "as to render Contagious Diseases very seldom infectious to different Species" (Bates 1718, 884). In his *A short discourse concerning pestilential contagion*, Mead seems skeptical that the French cattle disease will infect humans; he follows Bates in asserting that most plagues are "confined to a particular *Species*" of animals, and offers as an example the "Disease of the Black Cattle a few Years since, which neither proved infectious to other Brutes, nor to Men" (xxxii). Instead, Mead, a deeply committed iatrochemist (one who attributed disease and chemical reactions to the interaction of various sized particles), and a noted authority on poisons and snake venom, is markedly preoccupied with the contagious possibilities of "Goods"; he singles out cotton as the "most dangerous" for conveying the plague, and especially cotton imported from Turkey. In support of this argument, he recycles a story from Boccaccio's *Decameron* about "two *Hogs*" who found and ripped with their teeth the "*Rags*" (xxxii) from a man dead of the plague; both beasts died within the hour. Boccaccio's story, for Mead, justifies a prophylactic embargo on textiles. Mead's *Short discourse* ran through seven editions in a single year and led to a parliamentary committee whose remit was to recommend plague mitigation policies. The Quarantine Act of 1721 contained some familiar precautions—quarantines for incoming vessels and their crews, places for airing cargo to destroy or dissipate pathogens—and the authority to draw a *cordon sanitaire* around any infected town, halt commerce, and implement a death penalty for offenders (Mullet 1936, 488). The Quarantine Act explicitly covered both Great Britain and Ireland, along with the Channel islands of Guernsey, Jersey, Alderney, Sark, and Man. Three of these four British islands were known for their fine cattle breeds (Guernsey, Jersey, and Alderney, the latter now extinct), the Isle of Man for its sheep, and Ireland for its massive and by-now illegal imports of cattle through Scotland (Spinage 99). Arguably, the islands' inclusion in the Quarantine Act testifies to how critical they were deemed for England's food security.

The association between textiles—especially second-hand textiles—and disease, as Susan North argues, was a staple of early modern plague literature. Henry VII had issued the first official act regarding potentially contaminated bedding in 1495 (North 2020, 53–81). Wools and leathers were regarded as especially dangerous because the former, in the words of Stephen Bradwell, "retaineth the infection long," and the latter, "through their sponginess," do "drawe and keep it much more then other wearings" (Bradwell 1625, 18; see also Henderson 2023, 372–285). Mead's concerns about infected textiles, then, had a long history, one echoed by many of his contemporaries, including his friend, John Quincy, a noted apothecary. In his *Essay*, Quincy claims that the "Histories of Physick abound" with accounts of seemingly healthy people carrying "*Pestilential Miasmas*" (254–255) either in their clothes or in the goods they trade. Among these goods are cattle; Quincy mentions a "strange Story" about a "great Rot amongst sheep," brought into England by one infected sheep "bought for its uncommon Largeness" (256). It took fourteen years to root out this infection, he asserts. In his mind, these stories reinforce the "Prudence" of nations that impose immigration and trade regulations and that "enjoin all Persons and Merchandize from infected Countries, to stay a certain Time upon their Coasts and Borders before they are suffered to intermix with a healthful People; having by such Instances as here mentioned been justly alarmed at the Incroachment of such dreadful Destroyers" (255–56). Sounding much like Bradwell, Quincy insists that "nothing is more likely to preserve [the plague] than animal Substances, as Hair, Wool, Leather, Skins, *&c.* because the very Manner of its Production, and the Nature of its Origin, seems to give it a greater Affinity with such Substances than any other" (274). In such comments, the difference between live animals and animal products collapses under the language of plague mitigation and trade policy.

Although Quincy advocates quarantines of merchandise, he also takes up in a more systematic way than Mead the question of potential cross-species contagion, relying heavily on Lorenzo Bellini's mechanical account of the blood (English translation, 1720). For Bellini, the diseased body suffers from inefficient or imbalanced circulation, and particular diseases can be attributed to increased or diminished blood velocity (Bellini 1720, 155–57). Bellini, a physician and anatomist who wrote during Italy's cattle plague crisis, like Quincy, entertained the possibility of cross-species contagion. "If," as Quincy writes, "these subtile and active Particles [of contagion] be of that Nature, that they can penetrate the Pores of other Animals, and occasion a like Coagulation of their Blood,"

> not only Men, but Brutes also, will be seized with a *Pestilence*; but this does not always very necessarily happen, because the Blood of Animals is different from humane Blood, so that although these Particles are supposed to get into it, it does not necessarily follow that they must vitiate it, any more than will Aqua Regia dissolve all kinds of Metals; but yet Brutes of all kinds, or some of them only, will be seized equally with Men, when this subtile and active Ferment, which penetrates the Surface, is of that Nature, as will taint the Blood of other Animals with those *pestilential* Requisites. (263-64)

Using the language of iatrochemistry in ways that underscore uncertainty about what we now know as blood groups, and building his argument on "ifs," "yets," and "buts," Quincy creates a conceptual space for reverse zoonosis: when contagious "Particles" are "of that Nature" to "Taint the Blood of other Animals," he writes, "animals will be 'seized equally with Men'"; if infection does not always occur, this is only because "the Blood of Animals is different from humane Blood" (263). The contagion "Particles," in other words, may not always find a suitable host. Both Hodges and Quincy, in brief, acknowledge that animals suffer from diseases that, at least sometimes, can infect humans, and vice versa.

Corpuscular and iatrochemical accounts of cross-species contagion jostle with other theories that foregrounded insects, broadly imagined, as active agents of infection and transmission. In his *Plague*, Richard Bradley, a botanist, extrapolates from accounts of blight in plants and animals to sideline his contemporaries' fascination with blood and fevers. Relying on reports that "dead Bodies of the miserable People of Marseilles were found full of *Insects*" (41), he argues that plant blights and "epidemics in man and in animals, were caused by animalcules," which he sometimes referred to as "insects" or "worms" (Wilkinson 1992, 47). Bradley uses the plague at Marseilles, then, to yoke under one approach other seemingly insect-induced, multispecies mass mortality events, including the 1682 murrain on the borders of Italy that spread to Switzerland, noted in Chap. 2. This outbreak, he reports, "seem'd to propogate it self in the form of a *Blue Mist*" (21), killing most of the cattle in twenty-four hours; contemporaries, like Ludvig Holdberg (1684–54), described the blue mist as swarms of nearly invisible insects (Hünniger 2024, 89–90). Bradley emphasizes that those who managed the cattle "without a due respect to their own Health, were themselves Infected and Died away like Beasts" (21). In the same vein, he suggests that the "raging Distemper" of 1714, which reached within twenty miles of London, may have been insect related: "It was so Violent and Infectious, that if *one* [cow] had it, all others that came within Scent of her, or even eat where she Grazed, were surely infected; it seized their Heads, and was attended with running at the Nose, and a very nauseous Breath, which killed them in three or four Days" (28). The herdsmen, Bradley reports, blamed the contagion on the "unusual dry Summer, and the continued *East*-Winds," which he explains as follows: because the summer had been "extreamly dry, attended almost constantly with *Easterly* Winds," the ponds dried up, making it "probable" that "some Poisonous Insects were lodged and bred" (35). And because grazing pastures were "almost burnt up" and garden plants ravaged by insects, rendering them "unfit for Table Use," infested garden plants were "given to the Cattle" (35) who subsequently died.

Bradley's language of "worms," "insects," and "blights" may seem crude to modern epidemiologists, harking back to the rhetoric of locust infestations and disease that I discussed in Chap. 2. Yet as Melvin Santer notes, even though "no one in the early decades of the 18th C. could venture anything more than a philosophical speculation about the cause of infectious disease" (2009, 567), Bradley's bioenvironmental model admits the possibility of cross-species infections transmitted by a living agent. His belief in a contagious agent capable of reproduction—a *contagium animatum*—was shared by the French physician Jean Baptiste-Goiffon, who was charged by the French government with preventing the Marseilles plague from reaching Lyon (Wilkinson 1992, 48). As Dominik Hünniger argues, by the mid-eighteenth century, thanks to Antoni van Leeuwenhoeck and Nicolaas Hartsoeker, "insect theory" or a "microscopy of small organisms and cells would become one of the most influential explanatory models of cattle disease" (90), particularly in Germany. Such an approach recalls the rhetoric of *buprestis*, to be sure, but it also looks forward to later speculations about airborne viruses and to anthrax, whose causative agent (*bacillus anthracis*) produces spores that can remain in the soil for decades, then erupt under the right environmental conditions. If "India, China, South Africa, and America have no cattle plagues," Bradley maintains, then the murrains in western Europe offer "further proof" that "insects are the Cause of it, and that they are brought" from Asia, "with the Easterly Winds" (31). While Bradley sorely overestimates the ability of spores and viruses to travel long distances on winds, his insistence on biological agents of infection from the "East" nevertheless serves as a useful counterpoint to the equally speculative theories of natural philosophers and physicians like Hodges, Mead, and Quincy. Bradley assumes with many of his contemporaries—including Defoe—that cattle plagues may come from "Tartary," then spread into "Europe, Asia-Minor, Palestine, Barbary, and other South Coasts of the Mediterranean Sea without meeting anything in their Way to obstruct their Course" (38). Once again, Bradley's theory demonstrates how the Mediterranean cattle markets of Shakespeare's Venice, by the eighteenth century, had grown into a global livestock trade linking Western Europe and the steppes of Eurasia, both economically and epidemiologically.

Defoe and Flesh Markets

As in Shakespeare's Venice, fears about cattle plague often take the form of debates about tainted meat in metropolitan markets and the possibility that meat-eating could be one source of bubonic plague. Contending that corrupted meat was not plentiful enough to crowd the market and therefore "could not be supposed to extend to so universal an Effect" (59) Hodges, for one, remains skeptical about this explanation. Nonetheless, he includes tainted flesh in his list of potential causes of the plague as "the Opinion of Many," and acknowledges that in "the Year before the late pestilential Sickness,"

> there was a great Mortality amongst the Cattel, from a very wet Autumn, whereby their Carcases were sold amongst the ordinary People at a very mean Price; and a great deal of putrid humours in all likelihood produced from thence: And this, in the Opinion of many, was the Source of our last Calamities; and many knowing Persons ascribe the Pestilence to this Origin, as the morbid Disposition which such a Feeding must needs subject the people, could not but facilitate both the Infection and Progress of that Fatal Destroyer. (58–59)

Popular opinion about flesh from diseased animals giving rise to sudden outbreaks of endemic human disease persisted for two centuries. In such cases, theories of contagion morph into cautionary narratives about corrupted consumerism, with significant implications for public policy.

To offer one example, after the plague at Marseilles, Richard Blackmore, physician-in-ordinary to King William and a successful, if much-satirized poet, lists in *A discourse upon the plague, with a preparatory account of malignant fevers* (1721) potential causes of bubonic plague, including "unwholesome Meats and Drinks such as tainted and perishing Flesh" which, in times of dearth, "starving People greedily devour" (Blackmore 1721, 23). Probably borrowing from Girolamo Fracastoro, who argued in the sixteenth century that "plague seeds" could infect both humans and cattle, Blackmore holds that "Pestilential Atoms, which are the Seeds of the Plague," may be "communicated to the Body by Flesh…on which the infected Air has shed its Poison, which being admitted into the Stomach, affect the Spirits, and create Putrefaction in the Blood" (73–74; see Spinage 97). He then explicitly considers the relationship between cattle plague and bubonic plague, but only as part of an argument *against* the regulation of imported goods. Although "Murrain among Cattle of different Kinds," he claims, "is a Plague as contagious and destructive as the Pestilence among Men," both usually are produced by what he calls "Domestick Causes": "Murrain is bred at Home by unwholesome Herbs, bad Water, Malignant Air, &*c.* and is not deriv'd from Commerce maintain'd by Navigation with Foreign Countries" (27). A strong supporter of William and Mary in the 1690s, Blackmore here brandishes a Whiggish ideology, one intended to protect what later in the century would be known as "free trade." Pestilence is most prevalent, he maintains, in periods of "great Scarcity" when people are both most susceptible and most "compell'd to Eat unwholesome and corrupt Meats"; for him, "Famine"—not bad, imported meat—"is the Cause of Pestilence, as

Pestilence in its Turn produces Famine, which therefore are mutual Causes and Effusion of one another" (25). If famine and plague are the effect of scarcity, he reasons, disruptions of international trade will exacerbate rather than help solve the problem.

Defoe shared Blackmore's objections to trade regulations, his Protestant religious zeal, and his fears about infected flesh. Defoe's *Journal* is markedly concerned with the quality of meat and the potential for spreading disease.[5] Several passages focus on butchers and their tainted or contaminated products: the plague rages "so violently" among the "Butchers" and "Slaughter Houses" (Defoe 1722a, 92) that H. F., Defoe's narrator, prefers to go without eating meat. In the shambles near Newgate, two people fall dead, giving rise to the rumor that all the meat is "infected" (279); the meat at Whitechapel is so "dreadfully visited" that butchers begin to slaughter cattle elsewhere, then bring the meat "to Market upon Horses" (92). And people willing to venture to the shambles to buy meat will not "take it of the Butchers Hand," but "oft of the Hooks themselves" (93), a reaction that renders the butchers as suspected plague vectors. These examples share a reluctance to commit unequivocally to the theory that tainted meat spreads the plague, even as they register the kind of popular fears that, in one instance, "spoil'd the Market for two or three Days" (91). By recounting these rumors and noting market-adjacent or market-related deaths, Defoe reinforces the uncertainty about meat as a potential plague vector and manifests the caution about carcasses and butchers also evident in *Due Preparations*.

In *Due Preparations*, Defoe devotes a good deal of time and energy to a story about a St. Albans parish family who decided to shut themselves in to avoid the plague. The father "went to a Butcher in *Rotherhith*, [a borough of Southwark] none having yet died of the Plague on that Side of the Water; and here he caus'd three Fat Bullocks to be killed, and the Flesh Pickl'd and Barrel'd up, as if done for a Ship going on a long Voyage; likewise six Barrels of Pork for the same pretended Occasions" (1722b, 68–69). "Fresh" meat supposedly ensures minimal corruption; pickling prevents putrefaction; and the choice of market minimizes exposure to a

[5] The literature on *Journal of the Plague* Year is extensive. See Wall (1998: 164–77); McDowell (2006: 87–106); Seager (2008: 639–653); DeGabriele (2010: 1–23); Thompson (2013: 153–67); Payne (2014: 620–36); Lau (2016: 23–39); Taylor (2021: 399–420); Alff (2021: 625–43). See also the arguments in Novak (1962); Mayer (1997); Guilhamet (2010); and Napier (2016).

disease that could be lodged in the butcher himself. Immediately following this anecdote is another precautionary tale that gestures to what seems a nascent concept—or fear—of zoonotic transmission. Having written to several people in the country, the father "caus'd Twenty Flitches of Bacon to be sent him, some from one Place, some from another; so they did not come to him all together, nor above two or three from any particular Carrier" (69). Seeking multiple sources for bacon makes sense only if the father fears infection in and by pork whose origins he could not vet. In other words, the practice seems to suggest caution about local outbreaks of animal plagues. Rather than addressing this possibility directly, Defoe makes what, for him, is a characteristic recommendation: that people "alter their manner of Life," to "LIVE TEMPERATELY and Sparing," which includes eating "less Flesh, less Sauce, and less of the half Digested Juices and Gravies of their Meats…by which they are brought to Eat their Meat half Roasted and half Boil'd" (44). His admonition springs, in large measure, from the legitimate concern that heavy sauces could either disguise the taste of tainted meat or, as blood and gravies, could themselves be made of uncooked or undercooked offal.

In marked contrast to Blackmore, Bradley, Quincy, and Mead, Defoe does not address directly the raging cattle plagues, although he comes close in *Due Preparations.* In the context of comments about "French cruelty" he mentions potentially infected sheep. Five soldiers, enforcing a *cordon sanitaire* to keep livestock disease from spreading, were shot, complains Defoe: "for having persued two Sheep, to Kill them within the [quarantine] Lines, least they should get back and Infect the Country, so that the poor Men were Kill'd for their extraordinary dilligence in their Duty" (122). In Defoe's telling, the sheep may or may not have been infected and the men may or may not have contracted their disease; these specifics pale in relation to the bigger danger, the fatal consequences of the French quarantine. Aside from this nationalistic cautionary tale against quarantines, Defoe has little to say—at least directly—on the cattle plagues contemporary with his plague writings.

Making this comparative silence even more surprising, or perhaps symptomatic, is that Defoe, himself the son of a tallow chandler and butcher, probably knew more than many physicians and most of his readers about the cattle industry in England. In *A brief state of the inland or home trade, of England* (1730), he uses the cattle trade as an example of how commerce, ideally, should work:

> Our *Flesh-Meat;* the Cattle are first Bred, then Fed, then Driven to one Fair or Market, then to another, then Sold to the Butcher, and then to the Eater. In every one of those Circulating Removes, the Breeder, Feeder, Drover, Butcher, with their Cattle, Horses, Servants, and Families, are severally maintain'd by, and get a small Share of Profits from the Creature Sold; and which is at last charg'd upon, and return'd from the Price of the Meat when kill'd, and Bought by the Consumer. (1730, 8)

In this passage, Defoe describes an economy based on the rendered body of live animals in a series of "Circulating Removes." He names some of these "Removes" in *A Tour thro' the Whole Island of Great Britain*, singling out many places—Brecknockshire and Radnorshire in Wales, the meadows adjacent to Norwich and Yarmouth, Chesam, with the Vale of Aylesbury, Thrapstom among them—as noted for breeding and fattening cattle bound to London and other population centers (1724, 1: 57, 1: 268, 1: 203). *A Tour* also contains Defoe's lengthy paean to the cattle and flesh markets of London, which begins "That of *Smithfield* for Cattle is, without question, the greatest in the World: no Calculation of the Numbers of Horses, Oxen, Cows, Calves, Sheep, *&c.* can be made." He lists fifteen other "Flesh Markets," old and new, that "have such Numbers of Buyers, and such an infinite Quantity of Provisions of all Sorts, Flesh, Fish, and Fowl, that…no City in the World can equal them" (2: 140). Because poor roads and bridges make droving harder and animals tend to lose weight on such arduous journeys, he advocates for an improved infrastructure through which cattle can be moved efficiently, without "fatiguing, harassing, or sinking the Flesh of the Creatures, even in the Depth of Winter" (2: 252–253). This infrastructure was particularly important for London and its environs.

As we know from Thomas Almeroth-Williams, London's streets were filled with live animals more various and numerous than a reader might assume from Defoe's passing references to hogs, dogs, cats, tame pigeons, and horses in *Journal of the Plague Year*. Drawing on evidence from newspapers, insurance policies, poll books, and a variety of other records, Almeroth-Williams identifies 258 active cow-keepers in the city between 1730 and 1800 (2019, 103). Dairy herds fringed the city, pigs were still raised in closed yards in residential as well as commercial neighborhoods, and horses of various kinds provided energy for agriculture, small-scale production, and transportation, in addition to serving as sources of entertainment and (sometimes) meat. In 1725 at Smithfield, 76,531 cattle—what Almeroth-Williams calls "meat on the hoof"—were sold in the city square. By 1786, "this number had risen 41 per cent to 108,175" (103; see also Bierne 2013, 133–162).

In Defoe's *Journal*, readers get a glimpse of the teeming trade in animal flesh, partly through his inserting into his narrative the municipal "Orders for Cleansing and Keeping of the Streets Swept": "That the Laystalls be removed as far as may be out of the City, and common Passages, and that no Nightman or other be suffered to empty a Vault into any Garden near about the City" (54). The "laystall" is a term for cattle being held for the market; their dung—what was emptied from the "Vault"—was used as fertilizer. This particular injunction, then, guards against two sources of infection: potential cattle disease and the effluvia from cattle excrement. We also see fleeting signs of the cattle trade in Defoe's remarks about how "Slaughter-houses" empty offal into the "*Tide-Ditches*" flowing through London and into the Thames (Cole 2023, 513–526). In support of his contemporaries who argued that the plague is spread by smells, Defoe points to the open sewers that carry waste products from the markets, particularly on the south side of the Thames: "These filthy Places receive all the Sinks, Necessary-houses, and Drains from the Dye-houses, Wash-houses, Fell Mongers, Slaughter-houses and all kinds of Offensive Trades; they are continually full of Carrion, and the most odious of all offensive Stench proceeds from them" (29). On the basis of such passages, Christopher Loar argues convincingly that Defoe's plague writings offer "an emergent form of ecological thinking" and urban planning made possible and perhaps even necessary by contemporary disease theory (Loar 2019, 312).[6] From this perspective, Defoe shares with contemporary physicians and natural philosophers such as Thomas Sydenham, Mead, and Bradley, among others, an understanding that plague is at some level an environmental problem "produced by the weather (unfavorable winds or stagnant air), swarms of microscopic animals or particles, or some combination of the two" (Loar 2019, 37). Yet Defoe was not a fan of plague walls or shutting up houses and was interested less in etiological issues than in practical solutions—notably sewage systems to direct offal and human waste away from London through a network of sewers or ditches (Wall 1998, 164–177; Alff 2021, 625–43). Later in his career, in *The Complete English Tradesman* (1726), Defoe fantasizes about completely

[6] On the relationship between ecology and plague more generally, see Cole (2016, 1–80); and Barney and Scheck (2010: 1–22).

outsourcing the breeding of cattle for a growing English population to Scotland and Ireland, which would allow "all the lands in *England*" to "do little more than serve for gardens" for the English "and to feed their cows" (249). Defoe's vision of an improved England is based, then, on the unimpeded movement of healthy cattle from Ireland and Scotland (where they would be bred), to the English countryside (where they would be fattened), to cities (where they would be butchered and sold).

Although Defoe's plague texts have been celebrated for their realism, his treatment—or non-treatment—of live animals has had long-standing implications for our ability to read human and animal disease as part of complex ecological systems. Human safety in the throes of bubonic plague is clearly the focus in *Journal of the Plague Year*, but Defoe's near-erasure of live animals, notably livestock, from the novel helps reinforce the historically inaccurate perception that human plagues could be cordoned off materially and imaginatively from disease outbreaks among cattle. Having said that, at two crucial points in the novel Defoe mentions live cattle, seemingly in passing, but in ways that complicate his anthropocentric, market-driven perspective of London during the 1665 plague. He first refers to a group of people who, having fled the city for the countryside near Henalt Forest, were starving: they "suffered" such "great Extremities in the Woods and Fields" that they had turned outlaw, offering "many Violences to the County, robb'd and plunder'd, and kill'd Cattle and the like" (171). In the eighteenth century, killing cattle was considered theft and therefore carried significant penalties, including imprisonment and even death. Second, and more relevant to my argument, Defoe tells the story of a confined "Citizen" who, having broken out of his house at Aldersgate, heads to Islington, where he finally secures a garret room at an Inn called the "*Pyed Bull*," the other rooms having been let to "some Drovers being expected the next Day with Cattle" (85). The citizen dies in the house, and within the week fourteen more people succumb to the plague. The name of the inn—"the *Pyed Bull*"—suggests it is located along a popular droving route; Islington, later home to the Metropolitan Cattle Market, was the fattening site for animals on the journey from Scotland, and Aldersgate Street provided an access point to Smithfield (Champion 1995). In mentioning the anticipated drovers, Defoe gestures to London's place in a fragile live animal trade that sustained the urban population. Yet his solution to the problem of diseased flesh remains narrowly focused on individual caution, rather than on any public policies or epidemiological understanding: choose your butcher carefully, he suggests, cook your meat thoroughly, and—especially during plague outbreaks, eat "less Flesh." Such cautions encourage his readers to tread carefully in potentially infected metropolitan markets, I suggest, even as his earlier *Farther Adventures of Robinson Crusoe* displaces the threat of cattle disease and tainted meat from Smithfield onto the alien cultures and dietary practices of the nomadic herders of the steppes.

The Steppes and the "Siberian Pest"

Defoe's attitude toward suspected zoonotic outbreaks—one shared by many of his contemporaries—seems to have been "mitigate locally, blame globally," as in his always derogatory comments about "Tartars." Advocating for a moderate diet of well-cooked flesh in *Due Preparations*, Defoe decries,

> a most unaccountable Habit that we are brought to by our vitiated Appetites in this Nation, [is] to Eat our Flesh Meat, of which also we feed immoderately, almost Raw: Indeed, some People may be said to feed little different from the *Tartars*, who Eat their Horse-flesh Raw, if we were but to be seen by the People of any other Country how we Eat, especially our Wild Fowl, the Flesh scarce warm thro', and all the undigested Impurities of the Entrails and Inside of them serving for our Sauce. I say, when Strangers see us feeding thus, they must be allow'd to take us, as they do, to be, if not Canibals, yet a sort of People that have a canine Appetite. (44–45)

This depiction of the Tartar-like Englishmen as "canine," if not lupine, threatens to degrade them to bestial status. At stake in Defoe's comparison between England's shameful dietary habits and those of his imaginary Tartars—who, unlike his countrymen, eat "Horse-flesh"—is his commitment to reforming English manners, health, and decorum. "Foreign Countries," he insists, "describe our way of Feeding in *England*, and tell us we *Devour* our Meat, but do not Eat it; *viz.*: Devour it as the Beasts of Prey do their Meat with Blood running between our Teeth" (45). Defoe's revulsion at his countrymen's "way of feeding" is mediated through the peoples of the steppes. His affect opens up the text to a complex history of Western European perceptions of the indigenous peoples and cultures of Central Asia.

The steppes are an ecoregion characterized by grasslands without large forests except along rivers and the coasts of lakes. A 5000 mile long belt of grassland extending from Hungary in the West through Ukraine and Central Asia to Manchuria in the East, the steppes were home to nomadic populations and huge multispecies grazing operations, both differing in striking ways from Western European agricultural systems. In the 1940s, Owen Lattimore found that pastoralists in Xinjiang owned 11.7 million sheep, 1.55 million cattle, 870,000 horses, and 90,000 camels (1950, 155). Throughout the early modern period and into the eighteenth century, travelers called attention to the immense scale of Chinese and central and south Asian civilizations in ways that produced awe and anxiety for European readers (Markley 2006, 104–41; Perdue 2005). When Nicolaas Witsen, mayor of Amsterdam who had traveled to Moscow, published his map of Asia in 1691, the British Royal Society's then-president, Robert Southwell, wrote a letter comparing his travel to "*Tartary*" as "*Columbus* like, the Discovery of a New World," bringing "at least Tydings of those Parts, which, from the beginning, have layn in the Dark" (Fig. 4.1). Given the "impenetrable Deserts," "endless Boggs," "inaccessible Mountains," and "mighty Tracts" of "Tartary" whose hostile climates have condemned its inhabitants to "an everlasting Solitude," mapping this area, he continues, is "no less difficult then a Geographical Description of the Bottom of the Sea" (Southwell 1691, 492). Vast stretches of grasslands and forests from present-day Kazakhstan to Manchuria were largely unknown even to the Czars who claimed these lands as part of the Russian Empire and often fought border skirmishes with Chinese settlers expanding to the west (Perdue 2010, 341–356; Schlesinger 2017). Evert Isbrant Ides, the Czar's ambassador who traveled to Beijing on a diplomatic and fact-finding mission between 1692 and 1695, claims that Siberia can be "justly compared to a Terrestrial Paradise" (A2v). He takes note repeatedly of the minerals and woods that, potentially, could finance the settlement of these frontier regions, sometimes in ways that approach the sublime: he is forced to "pass over in silence" the "overflowing plenty of tame Cattle, and Animals, and the wonderful multiplicity of their kinds … as being beyond the reach of a Pen to express" (A3v). For western Europeans battling periodic outbreaks of cattle plague and the fluctuating costs of meat, this "overflowing plenty" of livestock indicated that traditional cattle driving routes from Hungary into Italy, the Germany states, and the Mediterranean could be expanded eastward.

Comparatively little about steppe cultures was familiar to the British, French, and Dutch, except perhaps a general perception that nomadic

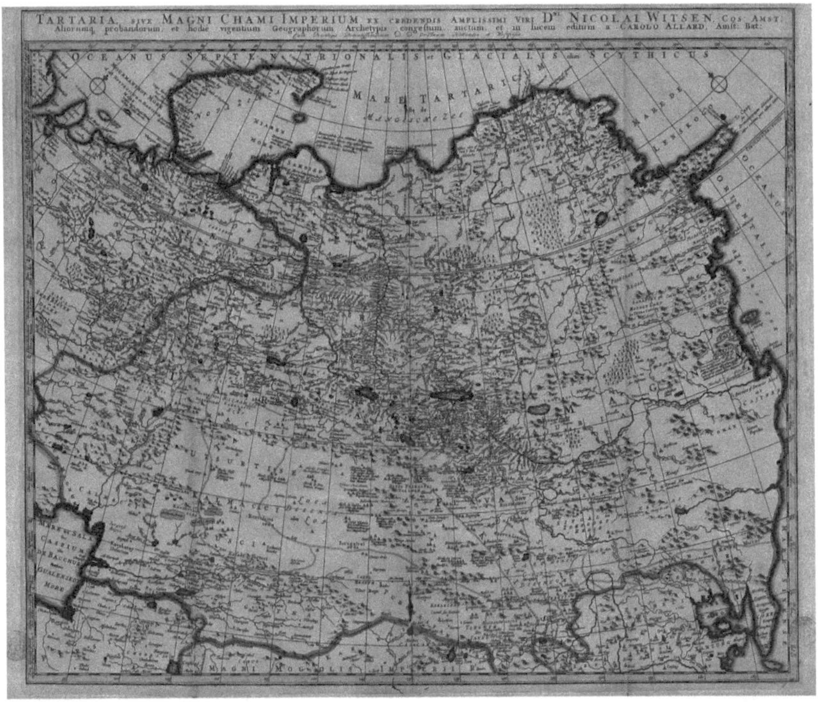

Fig. 4.1 *Tartaria, sive magni Chami Imperium ex credendis amplissimi viri.* Amsterdam, Carolo Allard, ca.1708. Biblioteca Nacional de Portugal

peoples were indifferent to western-style agriculture and their ways of raising and caring for livestock. Steppe cultures typically traveled with huge herds of sheep, cattle, and goats, consuming them along the way as need arose. These and other practices seemed alien to travelers like Ides. As Fernand Braudel argued half a century ago, "Europe chose wheat, which devours the soil and forces it to rest regularly"; because of this choice "Europe has always combined agriculture and animal husbandry" (Braudel 1977, 11–12). Livestock in England were pastured, counted, fattened, sheared, milked, sold, transported, and slaughtered, but the horses, camels, goats, and sheep of the steppes were described by eighteenth-century travelers and armchair geographers in ways that confounded a western European, Lockean understanding of property rights, agricultural improvement, and livestock management. Many steppe peoples grazed horses separately from cows, sheep, and goats because the latter eat grasses down to the roots, often damaging sensitive grasslands; by way of renewal, some nomadic tribes burned portions of the grasslands in order to produce early pasture for their cattle. Europeans—including Defoe in *Father Adventures*—sometimes mistakenly identified this practice as an act of aggression or war (Bell 1763, 1: 305). Moreover—again unlike the British—a significant part of their diet was composed of horses and horse milk.[7] Ides expresses surprise that "none of the Cows in Siberia and Daurai" who have suckling calves "will ever permit themselves to be milked"; "after the Calf is removed from them" their milk dries up, which is the reason why "Mares-Milk is so much used by these people" (44). These stubborn, unmilkable, agential cows are emblems of how alien the steppes are to Western Europe's agro-cultural practices. Although a vast resource for an expanding livestock trade, the Eurasian steppes were different enough to create fear.

The alien herding practices of the steppes seemingly made it easier for Defoe and other Western European writers to demonize the region for what became known as the "Siberian" disease, which most veterinary historians now believe to have been anthrax. Epidemiologically, anthrax, known under different names since ancient times, is endemic on all continents, except Antarctica. It is caused by *Bacillus anthracis*, a bacteria in the soil especially sensitive to variations in moisture, acidity, and humidity; modern scientists emphasize that the life cycles of this bacteria are influenced by climactic factors, such as ambient temperatures and precipitation (Ezhova et al. 2021, 217–228). Major epizootics of what likely was anthrax struck both people and different species of animals in Russia in 1309, 1374, 1375, 1443, and 1448.[8] Quarantines were introduced in the major ports of Italy as early as the mid-1350s. In the 1640s—two hundred years before it began to be known as "wool sorter's disease"—what we now recognize as anthrax was appearing regularly in the human population, so that a Czarist ukase prohibited the removal of skins from diseased animals and required that they be buried deep underground.[9] Although

[7] On the role of horses in Ottoman culture see Landry (2009) and Chaffetz (2024).

[8] See J. M. Koropov, *History of Veterinary Medicine in the USSR* (1954). Cited in S.G. Kolesov, "Anthrax." The only English translation is available in the Freedom of Information Act Electronic Reading Room. https://www.cia.gov/readingroom/document/cia-rdp82-00850r000300070003-8, accessed July 7, 2024.

[9] Kolesov, "Translation Anthrax." On Wool-sorter's disease in particular see Jones (2010: 2010) and Jones and Tiegan (2008: 455–485).

more common in warm climates, anthrax can survive in cold climates as well, and can be transmitted from cattle, whose grazing disrupts local soil ecologies, to humans, who handle skins or consume undercooked meat. By the late eighteenth century, commerce between Russia and Britain had grown significantly, and the earlier accounts by Ides and Bell had been supplemented by the works of later travelers, including Peter Simon Pallas: all became the basis for syncretic texts on Russia by reputable historians, like William Coxe (1780) and William Tooke (1799), both of whom spent time in St. Petersburg, as well as by popular compilers like John Trusler.[10]

Handling or consuming raw meat or skins is hardly special to the steppes, but as Russian exports of hides and cattle to western Europe grew in the seventeenth, eighteenth, and nineteenth centuries, so did reports of diseased livestock. The first recorded reference to what later became known as the "Siberian Pest," in Spinage's view, was probably a 1603 letter from a Russian ambassador who claims—"thank God"—there are now no more epidemics "among horses or men" (57). It was likely anthrax that spread through France in 1712 and was followed by bubonic plague at Marseilles. Nicolas Fournier, called upon to investigate the pestilence, recognized skin lesions that resembled plague buboes but were contagious in a different way; eventually he was able to distinguish clinically among anthrax, plague, smallpox, furuncles (boils), and scorpion bites (Swiderski 2004, 10). Ramazzini was the first European to distinguish between cattle plague (rinderpest) and the "carbuncular disease" (anthrax); the German botanist and geographer Johann Georg Gmelin described the latter, clearly zoonotic cattle disease, as the "Russian Disease," or "The Siberian Disease," in 1751 (Spinage, 57). Also in the mid-eighteenth century, the Russian physicians Abram Eshke and Plikita Nozhevshchikov were the first to note the latter's seasonality, and to link the symptoms of the disease in animals and people (Kolesov 1954). European scientists were unlikely to have had access to early Russian work; even now, it remains untranslated, and therefore accounts like Swiderski's *Anthrax: A History* (2004) begin with the Frenchmen Fournier.

Western views of "the Siberian Pest" remain deeply entangled with early descriptions of steppe peoples and their seemingly alien dietary practices, especially the practice of consuming diseased, undercooked, raw, or found—rather than domesticated—flesh (Trusler 1787, 2:300–324). Defoe's disgust in *Due Preparations* with "the *Tartars*, who Eat their

[10] On commercial relations between Russia and Britain, see Kaplan (1995).

Horse-flesh Raw" may have been triggered by Ides's account. Ides describes the "Samojedes" (probably Nenet people) "in Siberia" as "very like *Wolves* and *Dogs*, for they eat all manner of dead Carkasses, whether of Horses, Asses, Dogs or Cats, which die a natural death" (91). Even worse, he continues, they do not "take the trouble of dressing these Meats; but devour them raw":

> and if they had but Wings they would certainly take their flight to Greenland, and diet with the White Bears and Malmucks (a sort of Birds of Prey) which feed on the flead Whales Carkasses: And notwithstanding all this they inhabit a Country which richly abounds with Wild Game, Fish, and Flesh; but most of them are too idle to provide themselves with it. (91)

In this extended metaphor, the Russian steppe people are first compared to wolves and dogs, and then to bears and "Malmucks," or raptors (found in South Africa rather than Greenland). All the animals Ides mentions are apex predators whose prey fall in the wrong two corners of Levi-Strauss's cultural triangle: the raw, the cooked, and the rotten. John Bell, traveling through Siberia in the 1710s, took pains to combat Ides's negative stereotype, claiming that the Kalmyks eat horse meat broiled or roasted "and never eat it raw, as commonly believed, unless compelled by necessity" (Bell 1763, 1:34); the abjection of steppe people as less-than-human nevertheless persisted. Later in the eighteenth century, the botanist Pallas returned to Moscow from a six-year journey through Siberia, repeating the old claim that the "Kalmucks" (Kalmycks), Mongolic speakers residing west of Volga River, eat found and putrefying flesh: "Even the chiefs and first people among them . . . will feed upon cattle that have died of distemper and age, and let the flesh stink ever so much, they will eat it without disgust. For this reason, in every horde, the flesh-market has the appearance of a lay-stall of carrion" (Trusler, 2:218). This racist rhetoric attributes complex chains of infection to the adaptive cultural practices of nomadic peoples living in what, for Western Europeans, was an environment beyond the conceptual and cultural boundaries of Christendom.

The European treatises tend to both reveal and obscure what we now recognize as the etiology of anthrax infections. There are three types of anthrax—gastrointestinal anthrax, cutaneous anthrax, and inhalation anthrax, each spread in different ways. Given steppe ecology, meat was an essential part of the nomadic diet, and where there is meat, there is the threat of the first type of zoonosis: gastrointestinal anthrax. The climate on the western reaches of the steppe is defined by extreme seasonal variations. In the summer, temperatures have been recorded as high as 115 degrees F, and in the winter as low as –65 degrees F. These extremes necessitate seasonal dietary adaptations and raise the possibility of an increased likelihood for diseases of the digestive tract. Trusler makes the point that the Kalmycks "are never at a loss for meat in summer, as they can procure it in abundance, either by hunting, or from such of their cattle as die a natural or accidental death" (Trusler, 2:218–219). They eat wild horses, wild goats, wild boars, birds, badgers, marmots, and rats as "particular dainties" (219). During these summer periods of plenty, "they will cut [meat] into narrow slices, dry it in the sun or, in rainy weather, over a smoking fire within their tents, and lay it up for winter and travelling provisions" (219). But by the late eighteenth century, large swaths of the grasslands were already overgrazed or subject to overgrazing. Consequently, despite the huge sizes of the herds, cattle often died of disease, famine, or cold during the winter. Periods of scarcity affecting both cattle and humans were frequent.

Ides describes these hardships during a lean winter among the Kalmyks. Animals were rarely slaughtered, except by the wealthiest people, but scarcity forced change. As "soon as an Ox was killed," he reports, the Kalmyks "saved his Blood, and boiled it to the consistence of a Liver; this they eat instead of Bread" (86). No part of the animal goes to waste: "Others cut the Hides into slips, shed the Hair off, and toasted them at the Fire, and this passed at that time for good Food" (86). His qualifier "at that time" implies that the consumption of boiled blood and fired hides are adaptive practices, a way to forestall hunger and malnutrition in a harsh environment, when, during such lean times, no "part of the Entrails [were] thrown away" (86). Ides uses this description to link the Kalmyks to the equally disparaged black Africans: "had the scarcity [in Siberia] endured longer," he writes, "possibly [the Kalmyks'] Nature had been changed into that of *Caffers* or *Hottentots*, who not only eat raw Flesh but even the Excrements also" (86). As twenty-first-century readers, we recoil from these racist generalizations about central Asian and African peoples; at the same time, we need to see how fear motivated them, not only a fear of scarcity but also of disease. Eating undercooked or raw meat can lead to what Ides terms "inflammatory diseases," with symptoms including fever, chills, swelling of the neck and throat, painful swallowing, hoarseness, diarrhea, and abdominal swelling. All suggest the strong possibility of gastrointestinal anthrax.

Western European travel writers often describe what seems to them a different disease in Siberia that afflicts both humans and animals, likely cutaneous anthrax. One of the most detailed accounts in English is a translation of Pallas's German text that appeared in (slightly different forms) in Trusler's *The habitable world described*, as well as in the histories of Coxe and Tooke. While believing that the "chief ailment" of people on the steppes probably comes from "meat…eaten half rotten" (3: 129), Pallas (in Trusler's text) describes what he calls an "air-plague" raging in the area that had forced Russian authorities to institute a series of quarantines. Pallas had "difficulty" getting his horses into the fort, an "edict having been issued by the commanding-officer, that no strange cattle should be admitted into an infected place" (3: 131), although he eventually succeeded. "A description of this plague may be thought useless to an English reader," Trusler admits, "but when it is considered, that the same cause may operate in this and other countries, a little enquiry into it may not be unacceptable" (3: 131). His "little enquiry," following Pallas, runs several paragraphs—causes, symptoms, and cures. The symptoms of this disorder in humans include itching, "followed by a hard tumour in some particular part, which seems to arise from the sting of a fly, or horse-stinger" (3: 133). This swelling generally occurs on the face of humans (in horses, in the groin and abdomen) but can occur in any "uncovered" part:

> In the centre of this hard tumour is commonly discovered, in the external part, a red or bluish point, similar to the sting of an insect, and if remedies are not applied, the gangrenous putridity will extend itself farther. During this first stage of the evil, the patient feels no internal indisposition, but with the increase of the boil, he is afflicted with head-achs, anxiety and restlessness, which are, perhaps, but the natural consequences of his fear of danger; though the same anxiety, even to sadness, is visible in cattle but not till the distemper has reached it's highest degree and seems incurable. Some peasants, who accompanied me and had been afflicted with this disease, told me, that, after the first symptoms had shewn themselves, whenever they rode through a brook or within sight of water, they felt themselves very faint, feeble and ready to swoon. (133–34)

"Swooning" at the sight of water evokes traditional stories about rabies or hydrophobia—also a problem on the steppes—but the raised itchy bump that at first resembles an insect bite but then develops into a painless sore with a black center seems very much like the Mayo Clinic's description of cutaneous anthrax. As the sore swells ("with the increase of the boil") flu-like symptoms follow, including fever and "head-achs, anxiety and restlessness." In the acute stage for cattle and sheep, according to the Merck Veterinary Manual, abrupt fever "and a period of excitement" ("anxiety") is "followed by lethargy, stupor, respiratory or cardiac distress, staggering, seizures, and death."[11] Cattle, according to Pallas, "generally die of this distemper, partly because the boil is discovered too late, and partly because the common people do not like to meddle with the cows; but men presently get free from it, as soon as proper remedies are applied" (134–35). This, too, is accurate. In the absence of inoculation or post-infection care, cattle, sheep, and horses can die in two to three days.

Pallas also describes symptoms that may indicate a third kind of anthrax—infection through inhalation, what later became known as "wool sorter's disease." He terms this an "air plague" and attributes it to swarming "insects": in part because it seems to be related to "the hot summer-months," and especially "sultry south-winds," it "seems plain," he writes, that its "principal cause is certain insects hovering in the air, and almost invisible to the eye" (3: 132–33). Environmentally-generated insects might also explain, he continues, why the disease is less a problem in "towns or forts," why it primarily affects people "in the field, or when they go into the country, hay-making, attending their herds, &c. especially where the district is swampy" (3: 132). What he calls "air plague" is common among regiments on the steppes; when a "Kirguisian step" detachment passes such places in the night, writes Pallas, they "commonly" find dead horses the next day, and subsequently that the infection has "spread itself to men" (3: 132). Perhaps Pallas's description in Trusler's text conflates two kinds of anthrax in an effort to fit both under a single cause and to warn that Western Europeans may be subject to the same disease. While Pallas's insistence on "insects" as the source of disease aligns him with Bradley, who had imagined noxious insects carried from "Tartary" to "Barbary" on the wind, the German naturalist keeps open the possibility of more local and environmental conditions through which such "insects," or spores, could be awakened and dispersed. Taken together, eighteenth-century travel narratives about the steppes offer different etiologies of cattle and human disease—diet, air, insects—all made worse, presumably, by the region's extreme temperatures, its unhealthy swamps and forests, and the "savage" dietary customs of indigenous cultures. Despite pathological differences between anthrax and rinderpest, the steppes became, in the English imagination, the origin of pandemic cattle disease.

[11] https://www.merckvetmanual.com/generalized-conditions/anthrax/anthrax-in-animals#Epidemiology_v3271922, accessed September 25, 2023.

"Sinks and Receptacles of Filthiness"

Toward the end of *Farther Adventures*, the now 70-year-old Robinson Crusoe leaves behind the Great Wall of China with a caravan of merchants heading west across Siberia for Moscow. Crossing the disputed border between China and Russia, the caravan enters "the Muscovite dominions," and a city of "*Tartars* and *Russians* together, called Nortzinsky" (Defoe 2008, 192). Recent scholars have argued persuasively that Crusoe is embarked on an ideological mission to cast the "Tartars" as embodiments of savagery and paganism, most evident in his attacks on their idol-worship (Dharwadker 1998, 63–84; Markley 2006, 191–204). In one of the villages in the region, he comes "upon an old Stump of a Tree, an Idol made of Wood" that seems fashioned from the shreds and patches of a herding culture. The idol is "dressed up in the filthiest manner you could suppose; its upper Garment was of Sheep-Skins, with the Wool outward, a great *Tartar* Bonnet on the Head, with two Horns growing through it, it was about eight Foot high, yet had no Feet or Legs, or any other Proportion of Parts" (192). This diabolical idol—this "Block of shapeless Wood"—offends Crusoe's religious, cultural, and aesthetic beliefs, confirming his horror of pagan religions. "Sixteen or seventeen Creatures, whether Men or Women I could not tell," Crusoe tells his reader, "prostrate" themselves on the ground until he approaches them; then they "rais'd a howling Cry, as if it had been so many deep-mouth'd Hounds, and walk'd away, as if they were displeas'd at our disturbing them" (192). Crusoe assumes that the idol, known as Cham Chi-Thaungu, will be the scene of a sacrifice because, in a nearby hut "made of sheep and cow skins dried," he spots three sheep and a bull recently killed by three priests. "More mov'd at their Stupidity and brutish Worship of a Hobgoblin, than ever I was at any Thing in my Life" (192), Crusoe returns several days later, with two Scotsmen traveling with the caravan, to burn the idol while forcing its pagan priests to watch its destruction (Turley 2003, 3–20).

Defoe's over-the-top description of the Siberian idol as filthy, "brutish," and "sordid" (193) seems an elaboration—and degradation—of the household idols that Ides spots among the western steppe Ostiacks, who venerate "Gods made of Wood and Earth, in several humane shapes."[12] These idols, Ides observes, are dressed in "silken Cloaths, made after the

[12] This indigenous tribe probably was the Ket.

fashion of those of *Russia Women*" and "on the one side of the God hangs a bunch of humane and horse Hair" (19). The feminization of these idols appalls Ides and underscores his condemnation of this polygamous culture. "They call their God's Saitan," he continues, "and might indeed very well say Satan" (20). Ides is most offended by their method of honoring these objects, feeding them from "a wooden Vessel, with Milk Pap... [T]hey daily supply their Gods, and thrust it into their Mouths with a Spoon made for that purpose, but by reason that the Idols cannot swallow this milk Diet it runs out again at both sides of their Mouth, down their whole Bodies, in such a filthy manner as is sufficient to disgust one from eating of that Diet" (19–20). If he is recounting Ket practices, the "God" is likely a bear totem, who is treated as an honored guest in the hut. It may be no coincidence, then, that Ides gestures toward bears in a derisive story about how the Ostiacks mistake his "Nuremberg-Bear in clockwork" for a deity and offer to buy it from him (20). When worshipping or praying to this "nice God," he writes, derisively, they "chirrup or whistle through the Lips as we do when we call a Dog" (20). Significantly, in light of Defoe's *Farther Adventures*, Ides describes indigenous religious practices both as "filthy"—the only time he uses this word in his text—and widespread across "Tartary." Traveling to Surgut and to a people who similarly, in his words, have "no other Priests but their Conjurers," Ides once again details "wooden idols...which they feed as the *Osiaticks* do, with their best sort of Food, which runs out their Mouths over their Bodies" (31). Idolatry, filth, feeding practices that both horrify and amuse foreigners—all find their way into Defoe's depiction of Crusoe's "diabolical" wooden idol, destroyed by Crusoe in his self-anointed role as Protestant avenger.

Both Ides and Defoe, then, emphasize the combination of human and nonhuman cloths, hairs, and skins that adorn the Asiatic idols; the animalistic sounds of worship made by indigenous peoples; and the disgust, embodied in the word "filth," that this "Hobgoblin" arouses in them. Christopher Loar suggests that, for Defoe, Chaum Chi-Thaungu's "filthiness derives from its mixture of disparate animal qualities, the exaggerated size of its organs, and its lack of proper bodily integrity" (Loar 2014, 125). I would add that "filthiness" also implies disease, or the possibility of disease, both bodily and spiritual. In Defoe's fiction and nonfictional works, filth tends to be associated with feces, disembodied body parts, and hovering contagion. "Filthy," "filthiness," or its root "filth" appear eight times in *Due Preparations*, grouped into four passages. Two of these occur in Defoe's argument about how the "Bog-Houses and Kennels of the City" bring all the street "Filth" into the rivers, leaving behind "Carrion and Nastiness" when the tide ebbs (33). This emphasis on filth extends from animal excrement to abjected human bodies. The third instance is part of Defoe's argument that, at the beginning of a plague outbreak, all children from destitute families and in the workhouses be sent away, leaving London less encumbered with the "Poor, and with Children, and with all the Stench and Filth that attend those who want Conveniencies" and therefore would "Infect one another, and strengthen the Contagion in general" (24). The final reference in *Due Preparations* involves a mercury cure, often a dangerous treatment for venereal disease:

> All Sinks and Receptacles of Filthiness, say the Doctors, must be Cleans'd for the preserving our Healths, by sweetning the Air we breathe in; but what a Sink and Receptacle of Filth is the Body of Man? How is he to be restor'd but by Cleansing and Purging off the noxious Slime and Corroded Juices which are dispersed in all the Vessels of his Body, even those Vessels which common Catharticks will not reach. (41)

In "Sinks and Receptacles of Filthiness" Defoe includes a remarkable number of places: streets, rivers, workhouses, outhouses, animal yards, the scattered cottage industries about London, and finally the body itself. This is Defoe at the darker reaches of the Protestant imagination: physical corruption is both cause and effect of moral corruption.

Defoe's disgust with "the Body of Man"—"noxious Slime and Corroded Juices"—and with the unsanitary "Poor . . . who want Conveniencies" operates as a mode of abjection. As William Cohen writes, people "are denounced filthy when they are felt to be unassailably other…; actions, behaviors and ideas are filthy when they partake of the immoral, the inappropriate, the obscene" (Cohen and Johnson 2005, ix–x). Whether in relation to people or ideas, he continues, "all of these versions of filth have one thing in common: from the point of view of the one making the judgment, they serve to establish distinctions—'*That* is not me'" (x). Following the logic of abjection, if living in and around carrion and feces is more likely to be a problem with the English poor (which is why they must be evacuated from the city), the corruption of one's body through improper diet is more likely to be a problem of non-Christians, against whom the English must distinguish themselves. Defoe harangues his readers in *Due Preparations* that "if Men will meet an Infection with gross and foul Bodies, corrupted with the nauceious Fumes of ill digested Meats; with a Blood inflam'd with Excesses and Intemperance, whether of one sort or another…such Men may as well follow the Practice of the *Turks*, who, upon Principles of Prcdestination, Visit their Friends when the Plague is upon them" (42). The "vitiated Appetites" of England, especially the immoderate consumption of undercooked meat, threaten to reduce his countrymen to the level of the Islamic "*Turks*" or idol-worshipping nomads in Siberia. In his view, Eurocentric religious politics are tightly bound to the values and assumptions of cultural and agricultural existence—and to the disease policies that remain inseparable from Defoe's obsession with meat (Fig. 4.2).

In combining miasmic disease ecology with Christian moralism, *Farther Adventures* gestures to the threats posed by nomadic herds and alien

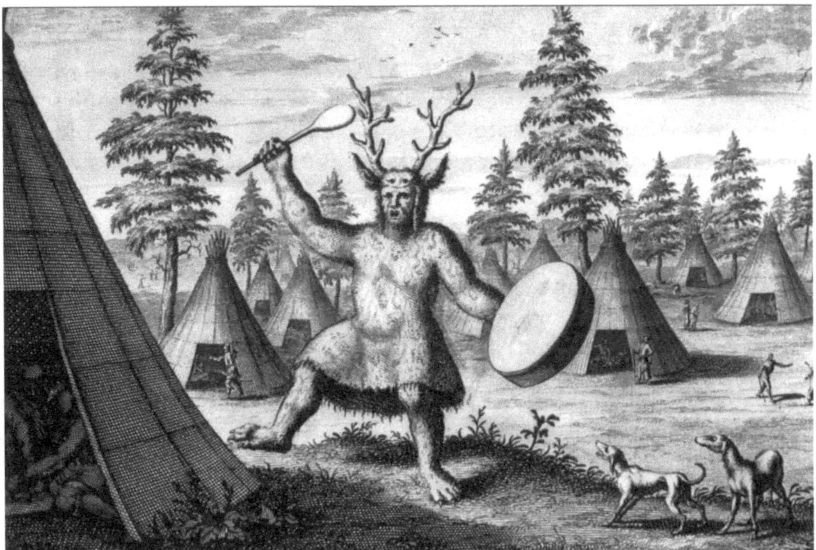

Fig. 4.2 *Een Schaman ofte Duyvel-priester*. [A shaman or Devil-priest in the country of the Tungus.] Nicolaes Witsen (1641–1717). *Noord an Oost Tartary* (Amsterdam, 1692; revised ed. Amsterdam, 1705)

peoples who, living outside the divinely sanctioned norms of property and European agriculture, threaten to consume Christian civilization and its avatars. In *A Vindication of the Press* (1718) Defoe declares that "Infidels possess such Vast Regions, and Religion in its Purity shines in a small Quarter of the Globe" (4). Destroying the idol, in this context, functions as what Defoe describes in *Due Preparations* as a mode of catharsis, a purgation—a "Cleansing and Purging of the noxious Slime and Corroded Juices" that, in his mind, are necessary to combat the threats of disease and idolatry. After smoking the priest and several other villagers out of their huts, Crusoe and his compatriots bind and gag them, then force them to watch as he and his comrades "daub'd [the idol] all over" with "Tar" and "Tallow mix'd with Brimstone" (196). In a sadistic simulacrum of the Ket ceremony of feeding, they "stopp'd [the idol's] Eyes and Ears and Mouth full of Gun-Powder, and then . . . wrapp'd up a great Piece of Wild-fire in his Bonnet," sticking into him "all the Combustibles" they could find (196–97). In rationalizing these violent and vaguely sexual acts, Crusoe offers a backstory from earlier in the novel: the aftermath of a battle with Carib warriors on "his" island. He calls the indigenous idol-worshippers "the most barbarous" of "all the *Heathens* and *Pagans*" he has encountered, "except only that they did not eat Men's Flesh, as our Savages of *America* did" (192). This invocation of cannibalism a half world away is ideologically revealing: the sight of the idol leads him to recall the trauma his men faced when seeing the mangled bodies of their comrades. This "Horror" generates fears about what might happen if the crew were to "fall into the Hands of those Creatures":

> [The Caribs] would not only kill them as Enemies, but kill them for Food, as we kill our Cattle. And they profess'd to me, that the Thoughts of being eaten up like Beef or Mutton, tho' it was suppos'd it was not to be till they were dead, had something in it so horrible, that it nauseated their very Stomachs, made them sick when they thought of it, and fill'd their Minds with such unusual Terror, that they were not themselves for some Weeks after. (44)

Crusoe imagines his men imagining themselves as livestock being consumed by "Savages," projecting their "unusual Terror" in the Caribbean onto the "barbarous" "Pagans" of the steppes. Their fears of becoming waste products, their flesh and organs making their way through the digestive systems of "Savages," becomes Crusoe's correlative for the imagined vengeance of the Siberians if he goes ahead with his plan to destroy their idol. The Scots merchant describes what happened to a "poor *Russian*" who interrupted their worship: he was lamed, shot with arrows, and then burned alive in an act of retribution befitting the values of "a Crew of Monsters" (194). Sanctioned by his Protestant zeal, Crusoe's burning of the idol nonetheless reflects his fear that haunts all instances of eating. As Jane Bennett puts it, "all bodies are shown to be but temporary congealments of a materiality that is a process of becoming, is hustle and flow punctuated by sedimentation and substance" (2010, 49). Crusoe's physical and moral disgust in the earlier scene on "his" island resolves itself on the steppes into a projected fantasy of ingestion. This fear of being eaten surfaces before Crusoe embarks on his caravan leaving China. Trying to escape Dutch ships in the China Sea, Crusoe compares the cannibals on "his" island favorably to the "inhuman Tortures and Barbarities" of the Dutch: "it were much more dreadful *to me at least*, to think of falling into these Mens Hands, than it ever was to think of being eaten by Men; for the Savages, give them their due, would not eat a Man till he was dead, and kill'd them first, as we do a Bullock; but that [the Dutch] had many Arts beyond the Cruelty of Death" (167). European trade rivalries, colonial conflicts in the Caribbean, and religious zealotry in Siberia are all cast in images of eating and being eaten, of "unusual Terror[s]" that threaten to turn western bodies into food, excrement, and filth. On the steppes, "Tartar" herds and herders resolve into one filthy "Sink," and Europeans into flesh to be consumed, like the carcasses hanging in London's butcher stalls.

In his anxiety about the "filthy" steppes, Defoe reinforces a discourse about human sin, medical knowledge, and the progress of civilization that vies with and sometimes displaces the biblical plagues of Egypt as the ur-source of human and livestock disease. In his *Animal Plagues: Their History, Nature, and Prevention* (1871, 1882), George Fleming reframes the "very grievous murrain, known as the 'Fifth Plague'," as a cautionary tale about anthrax and the nineteenth-century Sanitary movement (3).[13] Fleming's history of animal diseases begins "with the land of Egypt as the unenviable birth-place of plagues affecting the lower creatures, no less than mankind" (2). Initially, he naturalizes the Exodus account, describing how the flooding of the Nile and then the retreating waters leave

[13] Fleming was a noted veterinary surgeon and was elected vice president of Royal College of Veterinary Surgeons in 1867 and President in 1880–1884 and again in 1886–1887.

behind a "reeking morass," but then, deploying the colonial logic of European superiority, Fleming links this geo-environmental description to a geo-political denigration of Egyptian methods of farming and livestock management. Citing an account by M. Hamont, the director of Egypt's first veterinary school, he describes at length how dysentery affects cattle, sheep, horses, and men, especially among troop horses and regiments. The cattle are so "weak in constitution," Fleming recounts, that "men are harnessed to the plough and the cart, in order that the land may be, although imperfectly, cultivated, and some assistance obtained" (3). Even worse, the cattle frequently succumb to anthrax "which is enzootic and epizootic in Egypt," and often "carries them off" in "two, four, and six hours" (3). For Fleming, the diagnosis of widespread anthrax among livestock is based on the descriptions he has read of raised and irritated skin patches. The medico-theological confirmation of this diagnosis harks back to the biblical account that, in contrast to Egyptian herds, those of the Jews survived this plague unscathed. Israelite "flocks and herds escaped destruction," Fleming insists, as a consequence of *both* God's "miraculous intervention" *and* the ways that Jewish dietary practices anticipate Victorian conceptions of sanitation: the animals survive because of "the great care with which Moses inculcated upon that people the necessity for separating the clean from the unclean, the healthy from the diseased" (5). Put simply, Fleming co-opts Judaic dietary practices to reinforce late nineteenth-century conceptions about hygiene, health, germ theory, and imperial veterinary science.

Fleming's *Animal Plagues* demonstrates how the Exodus narrative could be deployed to advocate for the colonial imposition of sanitary measures on cultures across Asia and Africa: according to this logic, the domestication of animals is essential to "civilization," and civilization must be defined by normative, Western European standards of breeding and slaughter that need to be spread to the rest of the world. Later in *Animal Plagues*, Fleming quotes approvingly the remarks of Thomas William Atkinson (1858) on the "Steppes of Central Asia," which by that time was widely accepted not only as a petrie dish for the "Siberian pest" but also as the geographical source of rinderpest, then raging across several continents. Fleming himself traveled to central Asia and recounted his adventures and observations in *Travels on Horseback in Manchu Tartary* (1865), though he has comparatively little to say about disease in the almost 700 pages he devotes to his summer travels through Manchuria. Nonetheless, in *Animal Plagues*, the observations of Atkinson, Ides, Bell, Pallas, Coxe, and Tooke, among many others, are subsumed within a medico-ideological set of nineteenth values and assumptions. The patriarchal chiefs of these nomadic peoples, writes Atkinson, are surrounded by thousands of animals in a zoological Tower of Babel: "The screams of the camels, the bellowing of the bulls, the neighing of horses, and the bleating of sheeps and goats, formed a pastoral chorus such as I had never heard in Europe" (1858, 497). Fleming casts this "very Babel" (xviii) as an earlier state of human sociocultural and agricultural development surpassed by European civilization: "when a suitable and propitious locality has been found for their animals, the wandered perhaps become a settled people, and till the ground for themselves while still attending to the herds; and this combination of pursuits, which we term Agriculture, generally ensures a progressive and prosperous civilization" (xvii). While the biblical Tower of Babel explains the multiplicity of languages and cultures in the ancient world, the Exodus narrative, in this instance, offers a different kind of myth, one buttressing a Eurocentric theory of development: the cattle-grain system gives to rise to metropolitan settlement, and thus progress, prosperity, and the attendant values of western culture.

Nomadic peoples, Fleming asserts, have not yet fully embraced the grain and meat economies of European civilization—what he calls the "combination of pursuits, which we term Agriculture" (289). The inhabitants of the Asian steppes and their counterparts in other regions of the world must therefore be marked as the "wandered"—an archaic term, according to the OED, that applies *both* to humans and animals who "move hither and thither without fixed course or certain aim," and who are in motion "without control or direction." In the adjectival form, "wandered" creatures are "astray," or "bewildered," where "bewildered," literally, means lost in "pathless places" and, figuratively, mentally "confused." The "wandered," then, is a revealing locution because it signifies the not-quite-fully-human "others" of those agriculturalists who till the ground, pen the cattle, and enforce property boundaries so that fields and herds can be demarcated and claimed, owned by individuals, and nations.

If Defoe was aware of cattle murrains and steppe disease, such awareness, I have suggested, is largely displaced onto the nomadic peoples who live and sleep and clothe themselves with the skins of animals. Their habits paradoxically differ little from those of Robinson Crusoe in his goat skins. Crusoe wanders—and berates himself in *Farther Adventures* for his "chronical Distemper" (6) to travel the world—even as Defoe insists that he is not one of the "wandered," largely because of two practices. First,

Crusoe builds fences and cultivates small breeding operations, sacrificing raised animals to his own table. Second, rather than dressing wooden idols, he reads the Bible, reckons endlessly with the state of his soul, and casts himself as a Protestant Crusader (Hunter 1966). Ultimately, then, only ideological values and assumptions that link Christianity to European modes of agriculture and dietary practices distinguish Crusoe from the flesh-eating people he encounters, a difference reinforced through purposeful acts of violence against a "filthy" object. The fear and disgust that Chaum Chi-Thaungu provokes in Crusoe reminds him of his own animal body, the flesh-eating practices of Englishmen sickening themselves with undercooked meat, and the threat that contaminated flesh might be the zoonotic link between human and cattle plagues.

References

Alff, David. 2021. Make Way for Infrastructure. *Critical Inquiry* 47 (4): 625–643.

Almeroth-Williams, Thomas. 2019. *City of Beasts: How Animals Shaped Georgian London*. Manchester: Manchester University Press.

Atkinson, Thomas William. 1858. *Oriental and Western Siberia: Seven Years' Explorations and Adventures in Siberia, Mongolia, the Kirghis Steppes, Chinese Tartary, and Part of Central Asia*. London: Hurst and Blackett.

Barney, Richard, and Helene Scheck. 2010. Introduction: Early and Modern Biospheres. *Journal of Early Modern Cultural Studies* 10 (2): 1–22.

Bates, Thomas. 1718. A brief account of the contagious disease which raged among the milch cowes near London, in the year 1714. *The Philosophical Transactions of the Royal Society* 358:884.

Bell, John. 1763. *Travels from St. Petersburg in Russia, to diverse Parts of Asia*. Edinburgh: Robert and Andrew Foulis.

Bellini, Laurentius (Lorenzo). 1720. *A mechanical account of fevers*. London: A. Bell., J. Senex, W. Taylor, and J. Osborn.

Bennett, Jane. 2010. *Vibrant Matter: A Political Ecology of Things*. Durham: Duke University Press.

Bierne, Piers. 2013. Hogarth's Animals. *Journal of Animal Ethics* 3 (2): 133–162.

Blackmore, Richard. 1721. *A discourse upon the plague, with a preparatory account of malignant fevers*. London: John Clark.

Blagdon, Francis (trans.). 1802. *Travels through the southern provinces of the Russian Empire, in the Years 1793 and 1794, translated from the German of P.S. Pallas*. London: Longman and Rees.

Bradley, Richard. 1721. *The plague at Marseilles consider'd, with remarks upon the plague in general, shewing its cause and nature of infection*. 3rd ed. London: W. Mears.

Bradwell, Stephen. 1625. *A watch-man for the pest*. London: George Vincent.
Braudel, Fernand. 1977. *Afterthoughts on Material Civilization and Capitalism*. Translated by Patricia Ranum. Baltimore: Johns Hopkins University Press.
Broad, John. 1983. Cattle Plague in Eighteenth-Century England. *Agricultural History Review* 31 (2): 104–115.
Cavert, William. 2016. *The Smoke of London: Energy and Environment in the Early Modern City*. Cambridge: Cambridge University Press.
Chaffetz, David. 2024. *Raiders, Rulers, and Traders: The Horse and the Rise of Empires*. New York: Norton.
Champion, Justin. 1995. *London's Dreaded Visitation: The Social Geography of the Great Plague in 1665*. London: Centre for Metropolitan History.
Cohen, William A., and Ryan Johnson, eds. 2005. *Filth, Dirt, Disgust, and Modern Life*. Minneapolis: University of Minnesota Press.
Cole, Lucinda. 2016. *Imperfect Creatures: Vermin, Literature, and the Sciences of Life, 1600–1740*. Ann Arbor: University of Michigan Press.
Cole, Lucinda. 2023. Posthuman Ecologies. In *The Routledge Companion to Eighteenth-Century Literatures in English*, ed. Sara Eron, Nicole Aljoe, and Suvir Kaul, 513–526. London: Routledge.
Collins, Samuel. 1671. *The present state of Russia*. London: Dorman Newman.
Coxe, William. 1780. *Account of the Russian Discoveries between Asia and America. To Which are Added the Conquest of Siberia*. 3 vols. London: T. Strahan.
Debus, Allen. 1964. The Paracelsian Aerial Niter. *Isis* 55 (1): 43–61.
Defoe, Daniel. 1711. *The British Visions: Or, Isaac Bickerstaff, Sen. Being Twelve Prophecies for the Year 1711*. London: J. Baker.
Defoe, Daniel. 1718. *A Vindication of the Press*. London.
Defoe, Daniel. 1722a. *A Journal of the Plague Year*. London: E. Nutt, A. Dodd, and J. Graves.
Defoe, Daniel. 1722b. *Due Preparations for the Plague*. London: E. Matthews and J. Batley.
Defoe, Daniel. 1724. *A Tour thro' the Whole Island of Great Britain*. London: G. Strahan.
Defoe, Daniel. 1726. *The Complete English Tradesman*. London: George Ewing.
Defoe, Daniel. 1730. *A Brief State of the Inland or Home Trade of England*. London: Thomas Warner.
Defoe, Daniel. 2008. In *The Farther Adventures of Robinson Crusoe*, ed. W. R. Owens. London: Pickering & Chatto.
DeGabriele, Peter. 2010. Intimacy, Survival, and Resistance: Defoe's *A Journal of the Plague Year*. *ELH* 77:1–23.
Dharwadker, Aparna. 1998. Nation, Race, and the Ideology of Commerce in Defoe. *The Eighteenth Century: Theory and Interpretation* 39 (1): 163–184.
Eames, John, and John Martin. 1734. Experiments made with the bile of persons dead with the plague at Marseilles. In *The Philosophical Transactions (from the*

year 1719 to the year 1733) Abridged and Disposed under General Heads, 2 vols. 2: 595.

Ermus, Cindy. 2022. *The Great Plague Scare of 1720: Disaster and Diplomacy in the Eighteenth-Century Atlantic World*. Cambridge: Cambridge University Press.

Ezhova, E., et al. 2021. Climatic Factors Influencing the Anthrax Outbreak of 2016 in Siberia, Russia. *Ecohealth* 18 (2): 217–228.

Fleming, George. 1865. *Travels on horseback in Mantchu Tartary*. London: Spottiswoode.

Fleming, George. 1871. *Animal Plagues: Their History, Nature, and Prevention*. London: Chapman and Hall.

Franco, Guilano. 2020. The 1711 Rinderpest in Bernardino Ramazzini's XIII Oration and the COVID-19 Public Health Emergency: Facts and Common Aspects. *La Medicina del Lavoro: Work, Environment, and Health* 4:321–325.

Garcia, Humerto. 2010. A Hungarian Revolution in Restoration England: Henry Stubbe, Radical Islam, and the Rye House Plot. *The Eighteenth Century: Theory and Interpretation* 51 (1–2): 1–25.

Guilhamet, Leon. 2010. *Defoe and the Whig Novel: A Reading of the Major Fiction*. Newark, DE: University of Delaware Press.

Henderson, Stuart. 2023. The Organization and Output of the 'Controlled English Leather Economy', 1711–1830. *Historical Research* 96 (273): 372–385.

Hodges, Nathaniel. 1720. *Loimologia, or an historical account of the plague in London in 1665*. 2nd ed. 1721. London: Printed for E. Bell and J. Osborne.

Hünniger, Dominik. 2024. Bugs, Worms, and Dying Cattle: Multispecies Histories of Cattle Plague Outbreaks in the Long Eighteenth Century. In *Animals and Epidemics: Interspecies Entanglements in Historical Perspective*, ed. Axel C. Huntelmann, Christian Mieke Jaser, Roscher, and Nadir Weber, 85–94. Köln: Böhlau.

Hunter, J. Paul. 1966. *The Reluctant Pilgrim: Defoe's Emblematic Method and the Quest for Form in Robinson Crusoe*. Baltimore: Johns Hopkins University Press.

Ides, Evert Ysbrants. 1706. *Three years travels from Moscow over-land to China*. London: W. Freeman, J. Walthoe, T. Newborough, J. Nicholson, and R. Parker.

Jones, Susan D. 2010. *Death in a Small Package: A Short History of Anthrax*. Baltimore: Johns Hopkins University Press.

Jones, Susan D., and Phillip M. Tiegan. 2008. Anthrax in Transit: Practical Experience and Intellectual Exchange. *Isis* 99 (3): 455–485.

Kaplan, Herbert. 1995. *Russian Overseas Commerce with Great Britain during the Reign of Catherine II*. Philadelphia: American Philosophical Society.

Kolesov, S. G. *Anthrax*. https://www.cia.gov/readingroom/document/cia-rdp82-00850r000300070003-8.

Koropov, J. M. 1954. *History of Veterinary Medicine in the USSR*. Moscow, 1954.

Landry, Donna. 2009. *Noble Brutes: How Eastern Horses Transformed English Culture*. Baltimore: Johns Hopkins University Press.

Lattimore, Owen. 1950. *Pivot of Asia: Sinkiang and the Inner Asian Frontiers of China and Russia*. Boston: Little Brown.

Lau, Travis Chi Wing. 2016. Defoe before Immunity: A Prophylactic *Journal of the Plague Year*. *Digital Defoe* 8 (1): 22–39.

Loar, Christopher. 2014. *Political Magic: British Fictions of Savagery and Sovereignty, 1650–1750*. New York: Fordham University Press.

Loar, Christopher. 2019. Plague's Ecologies: Daniel Defoe and the Epidemic Constitution. *Eighteenth-Century Fiction* 32:31–53.

Markley, Robert. 2006. *The Far East and the English Imagination, 1600–1730*. Cambridge: Cambridge University Press.

Mascall, Leonard. 1578. *The first booke of cattell*. London: Iohn Wolfe.

Mayer, Robert. 1997. *History and the Early English Novel: Matters of Faction from Bacon to Defoe*. Cambridge: Cambridge University Press.

McDowell, Paula. 2006. Defoe and the Contagion of the Oral: Modeling Media Shift in *A Journal of the Plague Year*. *PMLA* 121:87–106.

Mead, Richard. 1720. *A short discourse concerning pestilential contagion*. London: Samuel Buckley and Ralph Smith.

Mullet, Charles. 1936. The English Plague Scare of 1720–23. *Osiris* 2:484–516.

Mullet, Charles. 1946. The Cattle Distemper in Mid-Eighteenth-Century England. *Agricultural History* 20 (3): 144–165.

Napier, Elizabeth. 2016. *Defoe's Major Fiction: Accounting for the Self*. Newark, DE: University of Delaware Press.

North, Susan. 2020. *Sweet and Clean? Bodies and Clothes in Early Modern England*. Oxford: Oxford University Press.

Novak, Maximillian. 1962. *Economics and the Fiction of Daniel Defoe*. Berkeley: University of California Press.

Payne, Geoffrey. 2014. Distemper, Scourge, Invader: Discourse and Plague in Defoe's *A Journal of the Plague Year*. *English Studies* 95 (5–6): 620–636.

Perdue, Peter. 2005. *China Marches West: The Qing Conquest of Central Eurasia*. Cambridge, MA: Harvard University Press.

Perdue, Peter. 2010. Boundaries and Trade in the Early Modern World: Negotiations at Nerchinsk and Beijing. *Eighteenth-Century Studies* 43 (3): 341–356.

Quincy, John. 1720 (rpt 1721). *An essay on the different causes of pestilential diseases, and how they became contagious*. London: E. Bell and J. Osborne.

Santer, Melvin. 2009. Richard Bradley: A Unified, Living Agent Theory of the Cause of Infectious Diseases of Plants, Animals, and Humans in the First Decades of the 18th Century. *Perspectives in Biology and Medicine* 52 (4): 566–578.

Schlesinger, Jonathan. 2017. *A World Trimmed with Fur: Wild Things, Pristine Places, and the Natural Fringes of Qing Rule*. Stanford: Stanford University Press.

Seager, Nicholas. 2008. Lies, Damned Lies, and Statistics: Epistemology and Fiction in Defoe's *A Journal of the Plague Year*. *Modern Language Review* 103 (3): 639–653.

Southwell, Robert. 1691. An Account of a Large and Curious Map of the Great Tartary, Lately Published in Holland, by Mr. Nicholas Witsen, being an Extract of a Letter from the Author Thereof, to the Honourable Sit Robert Southwell Knt. and President of the Royal Society. *Philosophical Transactions* 17 (193): 492.

Spinage, Clive. 2003. *Cattle Plague: A History*. New York: Kluwer Academic/ Plenum Publishers.

Swiderski, Richard. 2004. *Anthrax: A History*. Jefferson, NC: MacFarland.

Taylor, Jonathan. 2021. 'Books Frighted Them Terrible': The Perils of Propagating Fear and the Ethics of Writing about Disease in Defoe's *A Journal of the Plague Year*. *Literature and Medicine* 39 (2): 399–420.

Thompson, Helen. 2013. 'It was Impossible to Know These People': Secondary Qualities and the Form of Character in Defoe's *A Journal of the Plague Year*. *The Eighteenth Century: Theory and Interpretation* 54 (2): 153–167.

Tooke, William. 1799. *View of the Russian Empire during the reign of Catharine the Second, and to the close of the present century*, 3 vols. London: Longman and Rees.

Trusler, John. 1787. *The habitable world described, or the present state of the people in all parts of the globe, from north to south*, vol. 3. London: printed for the author.

Turley, Hans. 2003. The Sublimation of Desire to Apocalyptic Passion in Defoe's Crusoe Trilogy. In *Imperial Desire: Dissident Sexualities and Colonial Literature*, ed. Philip Holden and Richard J. Ruppel, 3–20. Minneapolis: University of Minnesota Press.

Wall, Cynthia. 1998. Novel Streets: The Rebuilding of London and Defoe's *A Journal of the Plague Year*. *Studies in the Novel* 30 (2): 164–177.

Wilkinson, Lise. 1984. Rinderpest and Mainstream Infectious Disease Concepts in the Eighteenth Century. *Medical History* 28:129–150.

Wilkinson, Lise. 1992. *Animals and Epidemics: An Introduction to the History of Comparative Medicine*. Cambridge: Cambridge University Press.

Williamson, Raymond. 1958. The Plague of Marseilles and the Experiments of Professor Anton Deidier on its Transmission. *Medical History* 2 (4): 237–252.

CHAPTER 5

1740–1790: Bovine Elegies and Bioinsecurities

Abstract By the mid-eighteenth century, cattle plague had become endemic in the Netherlands, and threatened to again infect herds in England. Robert Dossie's influential *Memoirs of Agriculture, and Other Oeconomical Arts* published in 1768 treats cattle plague as a "very momentous national evil" against which the government must provide "a means of security". This chapter returns to the issue of ecological vulnerability raised by *De Mortibus Boum*; it analyzes hymns, sermons, topical poetry, newspapers, natural histories, and eighteenth-century versions of the "bovine elegy," all of which reveal confusion, distress, and what we might now call bioinsecurity for the government and rural economies. Dossie was one of many agricultural writers who, partly out of desperation, partly driven by a desire to cut economic losses, began to question the efficacy of cull and bury policies, a long-standing tool of government plague containment and control. He argues that cattle plague is seasonal and therefore partly subject to the ministrations of good husbandry. While his turn away from cull to cure might be perceived as a sign of increased concern about animal welfare, I treat it as the paradoxical capture of cattle within an instrumental medico-economic regime. Separated from "Nature" in the public imagination, while still serving as disease vectors and victims, dying cattle provoked complex responses, from satire to affective, elegiac compassion. The chapter ends by considering the possibility that eighteenth-century eco-anxiety includes not only climate-related disaster but the trauma of mass animal die-offs.

L. Cole, *The Fifth Plague*, Palgrave Studies in Animals and Literature, https://doi.org/10.1007/978-3-031-92793-5_5

The distemper becomes the national habit.
Edmund Burke, *Thoughts on the cause of the present discontents* (1770)

The Dutch artist Jan Smit provides one of the few, and most widely circulated, visual images of rinderpest in the eighteenth century (Fig. 5.1). Rinderpest entered Holland in 1744 and lasted for about twenty years, resulting in the death of an estimated one million animals (Faber 1962, 1–7; Koolmees 2010, 19–41). The first thing one notes in this print, not surprisingly, is the scale of mortality. I count over fifty animals located in discrete pastures, most of them downed or dead. The number of expiring or belly-up cows, though, makes it easy to overlook other vignettes. To the right an official (or possibly a landowner), his right hand raised, seems to be giving orders or trying to still the panic, and to the left, in a scene replicated elsewhere in the image, people stand over or dig a grave. In the funerary scene closest to the viewer, another official appears to be exhorting the couple to throw a flayed hide into the mass burial pit. Several vignettes suggest failed

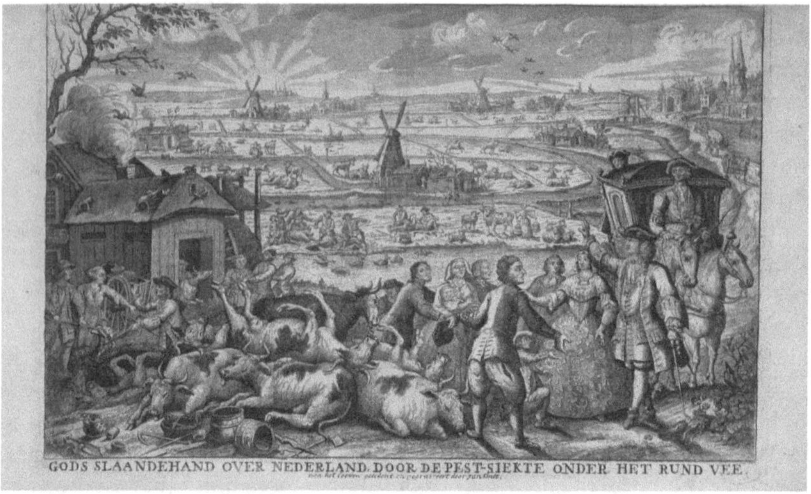

Fig. 5.1 Jan Smit, *Gods Slaandehand Over Nederland Door De Pest-Siekte Onder Het Rund Vee* [God's Punishment on the Netherlands Through the Cattle Plague]. 1745. Rijksmuseum Amsterdam. Public domain

cures. Behind the funerary scene is one of several smoking barns that either evoke fumigation, a common but ineffectual remedy for cattle plague, or the often-proscribed burning of hay in the vacated stalls of infected cattle. Pots and hooks strewn about suggest other desperate measures: some burned or ingested mixture of sulfur, tobacco-water, or gunpowder, all of which had been used as human preventatives against bubonic plague, and all of which, according to Robert Dossie, "do more harm than good" (Dossie 1771, 2: 390). The afflicted cow being dragged from the barn dramatizes why Daniel Peter Layard's *An essay on the nature, causes, and cure of the contagious distemper among the horned cattle in these kingdoms* (1770) begins with an apology. "To discover and account for the nature of the distemper among the horned cattle," he writes, "after it has raged for so many years in different parts of EUROPE, and moreover to ascertain a method of cure, appears at this time as difficult and unpromising a task, as it was of old to untie the gordian knot" (1770, 1). The cow being dragged off, presumably to be killed, serves as an apt image for the suffering and despair shared by the animals and the farmers alike.

The title of Smit's print invokes the scourge logic I discussed in Chap. 1, the belief that cattle plague is, as the title states, "God's Punishment on the Netherlands Through the Cattle Plague." Shortly after falling on Holland, in 1745 rinderpest re-entered England. It dragged on in both countries for a decade, waned, then broke out again in the 1760s. Smit's illustration implies a national calamity in the Netherlands, an epizootic so destructive, so uncontrollable, that its mortality rates provoked fears in Great Britain of a similar impending national disaster. In the words of one historian, the outbreaks in the 1740s and 1760s were "important enough in the government's collective mind, to vie with the '45 rebellion in Privy Council discussions in the autumn and winter of 1745–46, and to provide the opening item for the King's speech to Parliament in January 1770" (Broad 1983, 106, 107). The King's Speech to Parliament in March 1745, published in the *London Gazette*, is markedly pessimistic about the possibility of cure: "the Methods of Cure which have been put in practice, at Home and Abroad," George II declares, "have proved so unsuccessful, that they have rather contributed to propagate than stop the Infection; for while Means are used to save the Sick, the Disease spreads amongst the Sound, and is increasing more and more" (*Gazette* 1745). Although according to Lise Wilkinson, by the early eighteenth century some physicians had "a firm grip on the basic elements of epidemiology" (Wilkinson 1992, 41)—that is, on the containment of contagious diseases, largely through quarantining and culling—the seemingly unending disaster in the Netherlands made clear the limits of this necropolitical strategy.

This chapter investigates what it meant, during England's second and third rinderpest outbreaks, to face mass mortalities caused by a disease "no medicines can cure." Characterizing the nature, effect, and import of these mid- and late-eighteenth-century outbreaks of rinderpest and other afflictions, however, is not a straightforward task. Although eighteenth-century accounts of cattle plague and governmental responses seem plentiful in comparison to the early modern period, with which I began this study, their number is dwarfed by the volume of newspaper reports, religious texts, medical treatises, and policy documents generated during and after the 1865 rinderpest outbreak in England. This difference has led Harriet Ritvo to distinguish between the panic of the Victorian outbreaks—the subject of my next chapter—during which over half a million animals died, and what she regards as the lower-profile responses to the eighteenth-century epizootics. In the nineteenth century, she claims, both "the magnitude of the resulting economic disaster and fears for the soundness of the food supply prompted widespread concern"; in contrast, although the "rhetoric" may have been similar during eighteenth-century outbreaks, "worry about its causes and effects was usually short-lived" so that, "once over, even a catastrophic visitation left few traces in public consciousness" (Ritvo 1989, 167, 165). In one important sense, Ritvo is correct. Eighteenth-century outbreaks probably left less direct evidence in the "nonspecialist" historical record than did the great British outbreak of 1865. Yet "public consciousness" is notoriously difficult to locate. Before the histories of contagious diseases published by Noah Webster in 1799 and George Fleming in 1871, references to cattle plagues in England are deeply entangled, as we have seen, with a range of other discourses—theology, agricultural improvement, international trade, entomology, politics, nationalism, literature, and the local economics of plague policies. Clive Spinage offers the example of a 1717 satire accusing farmers ("cunning huxters") of killing their own old or lean cattle not because they were diseased, but in order to receive the compensation: "For every cow of Heaven's killing—/ A gen'rous bounty, that destroy'd/ More cattle than the plague annoy'd" (Spinage 2003, 114). The satiric targets, in this instance, are both farmers presumably gaming the system and the unintended consequences of a "gen'rous" government "bounty" designed, however inefficiently, to stop the spread of cattle plague.

Having said that, I doubt we have thoroughly investigated the varied effects of these repeated epizooties, the nature and contours of "worry" that outbreaks provoked. The King's 1745 Speech and the accompanying parliamentary orders, like the earlier mitigation measures on which they were based, signal a broad concern with what we now call biosecurity—the detection, surveillance, and containment of harmful organisms. Government infrastructure is intended to provoke a sense of preparedness—recall Defoe's title, *Due Preparations for the Plague*—but, as a recent study claims, such modes of governance simultaneously symptomize (and sometimes generate) bio*in*security, or vulnerabilities not shared equally by all members of a population (Chen and Sharp 2014). During COVID-19, "vulnerability" was used to mark groups of people differentially exposed to risk, generally but not always the elderly, those with co-morbidities, homeless or underhoused people, those in highly dense communities without proper nutrition or sanitation. Similarly, in the eighteenth century, plagues and diseases, climatic disruptions, local food shortages, and enforced culls affected differently situated members of the community in radically different ways. Smit's image of cattle plague in the Netherlands offers a marked contrast between the farmers and cottagers pleading in the foreground—distressed, anxious, grieving, afraid—and the well-dressed gentleman on the right. Rural laborers suffer more—or more explicitly—than those either issuing orders or expressing the eighteenth-century equivalent of their thoughts and prayers. Insofar as "vulnerability," unlike "panic," describes differential exposure to, and effects of, epidemiological events and the measures deployed to contain them, it provides a useful starting point for considering how affect is registered in the historical record.

The first section of this chapter hearkens back to *De Mortibus Boum* (Chap. 1) and to its Virgilian images of suffering cattle; it includes William Dodd's "Diggon Davy's resolution on the death of his last cow: A pastoral," published, in part, by Edward Cave in the *Gentleman's Magazine* during the 1740s enzootic, then in full after Dodd's death (Dodd 1767, 260–264).[1] Dodd (1729–1777), once a popular parson in Bloomsbury, wrote some fifty-five works during his lifetime, which more or less coincided with England's rinderpest outbreaks. That Dodd, nicknamed "The Macaroni Parson," was hanged for forgery (against the objections of Samuel Johnson) has made him something of a joke, but his "Diggon Davy," together with similar poems and hymns, is representative of what I call the "bovine elegy," a sub-genre of the georgic that appeared with some frequency during these mid-century outbreaks. Perhaps given a still-active tradition of pastoral care in agricultural regions, perhaps because rural people and their animals were so interdependent, images of dead and

[1] See Barker (1982) on Dodd's verse.

dying cattle played an outsized role in homiletic and devotional literature written by and for farmers and members of farming communities. These bovine elegies, much like the many cattle-themed hymns and prayers for livestock emerging from the pulpit, attest to both a growing impatience with blanket culling policies and a first-hand knowledge of—and sympathy for—dying animals. For a significant number of writers and their audiences, images of dying and suffering cows helped to consolidate opposition to what was increasingly perceived as governmental interference and ineptitude, a frustration culminating in the 1770s. Such images, literary or visual, like Smit's, also offer a corrective to the historical record. As Joseph Hardwick recently has argued, historians have mostly focused on the effects of cattle plague from one of three perspectives: the veterinary profession, the development of germ theory, and animal disease control, or policies, including mandatory culls. "Little," he claims, "has been written on how communities understood or reacted to the suffering of cows" or how—especially within religious circles—mass mortalities manifested in feelings that "the human relationship with the natural world was somehow wrong and broken" (Hardwick 2024, 154–55). For Hardwick, such concerns can be read as an early form of "ecological thinking" (156).

The second section focuses on the work of the chemist Robert Dossie (1717–1777), whose influential *Memoirs of Agriculture, and other Œconomical Arts*, published during England's third eighteenth-century outbreak, treats cattle plague as a "very momentous national evil" against which Great Britain must provide "a means of security" (367). Describing in detail the devastation of cattle in the Netherlands, he insists "what happened there ought to be an object of dread, as well as our compassion" (481). It therefore

> behoves every individual to exert his utmost endeavors, according to his situation, to avert this impending danger of one of the most heavy calamities that can befall any European country: and more especially our own; where the luxurious habits of the common people, the difficulty of obtaining a supply of cattle from other places, and the high process of the necessaries of life, would render the effects of a scarcity of horned beasts, and consequently all other provisions, peculiarly grievous and intolerable. (482)

Although Dossie gestures toward scourge logic in his comment about "the luxurious habits of the common people" (they eat too much meat), he combines the language of sensibility—"compassion"—with Defoe's keen emphasis on economics, primarily the importance of the cattle trade, the food and labor shortages cattle plague can produce, and the fear that bad or misguided policies can exacerbate food scarcity. Citing substantial evidence from physicians in the Netherlands, Dossie is perhaps the first person to lay out in systematic epidemiological and economic terms the problem with any blanket stamp-out policy: in his argument, it overestimates the ability of both farmers and officials to know if an animal is sick and must be killed, and it miscalculates the cost of keeping an exposed animal alive. As we shall see, Dossie argues for a more nuanced, necropolitical approach to murrain than did his predecessors, the early eighteenth-century Italians and their English counterparts. He resists traditional policies—quarantine, cull, and bury—by trying to establish empirically that cattle plague is seasonal, primarily related to cold, its morbidity rate dependent on the constitution and treatment of individual animals. In effect, he argues that cattle share with humans an "epidemic constitution." In ways that are too familiar to both farmers (and some pet owners), Dossie makes clear that, in the face of disease, cattle must be treated as pathologized individuals, rather than as part of a herd—this, even as he calculates value of individual animals down to the pence.

Read together, these sections—one focused on compassion for dying cows and their people, the other on plague mitigation during the "age of sensibility"—illustrate close, if sometimes contradictory, relationships among disparate discourses and practices: ecological thinking, national and local economics, care for suffering animals, and a rapidly developing plague bureaucracy. As Nicolo Paolo Ludovice puts it, epizootic outbreaks "unravel relationships that were often glossed over in history"; to focus on government policy, on "disease control missions" (Ludovice 2021, 6), without also attending to the complex relationships between humans and animals simply reinforces this problem. Recent scholarly efforts to complicate a narrow focus on policy apart from complex interactions between animals and people include Ludovice's own work on rinderpest in the Philippines and Indochina, Natalie Porter's study of bird flu in Vietnam, and, in different ways, the foundational collection *Healing the Herds: Disease, Livestock, and the Globalization of Veterinary Medicine* (Ludovice 2021; Porter 2019; Brown and Gilfoyle 2010). This chapter is intended to open—or to *re*open—a conversation about sensibility, the multispecies nature of great mortalities, and their differential effects in eighteenth-century England. "Bioinsecurity"—which includes its cousin, "eco-anxiety"—is the umbrella term under which, I argue, large-scale catastrophes, small-scale intimacies, and epizootic outbreaks can be considered as related phenomena.

The Bovine Elegy

On March 12, 1745, King George II announced an Act of Parliament that allowed the sovereign to pass orders and laws to "more effectually prevent the spreading of the Distemper which now rages among the Horned Cattle in this Kingdom" (*Gazette* 1745, 10). Resurrecting a dormant network of Justices of the Peace, various legal officials, informers, inspectors, ministers, physicians, and houses of correction, these orders were to be read every Sunday after prayers as long as they were in force. They restored the quarantine and cull policies of the 1711–1714 outbreak: when cattle appear to have "Signs or Marks" of the distemper, they must be separated from the herd and "shot dead, or otherwise killed" while spilling as little blood as possible; hides should be slashed "from Head to Tail" (10–11) to prevent them being sold, the body buried at least four feet deep. The remaining six orders, according to John Broad, "revive the 1714 regulations almost word for word" (1983, 106–107). They mandate cleaning and fumigation of stalls and cattle; prohibit selling infected meat or using it as livestock feed; establish the length of quarantine (one month); and require reports to and from constables, churchwardens, parish overseers, and appointed inspectors about any infected cattle. These designated officials, moreover, were required to meet with Justices "from time to time" to "hear complaints," "punish Offenders," and convey to the Privy Council an "exact account" (11) of mortality rates and what they have done to stop the spread of disease. By way of "Encouragement" to farmers whose cattle have caught the disease, the Treasury promises to pay half the animal's value for every culled cow or bull, not to exceed the "Sum of Forty Shillings," and a quarter of that for calves, so long as the "infected Beasts" were "shot, or otherwise killed, slashed, and buried according to the above Regulations" (12). Published in the *London Gazette*, these orders were to be updated annually over the next decade. For the next two years, however, the movement of cattle out of any town or parish "to any Fair, Market, or any Other Town" was prohibited or regulated for specified periods of times, allowed again only on the condition that cattle had been certified as having a clean bill of health (*Gazette* 1746). Subsequent orders extended these prohibitions nationwide and provided more specifics, including mounting a list of infected places in a prominent site on every

High Road. In brief, as Broad argues, the 1745 orders created a "fast multiplying plague bureaucracy" (107) fraught with logistical difficulties, evasion, and corruption.

The officials tasked with enforcing these orders, significantly, included not only constables, justices of the peace, and parish overseers, but also "the Overseers of the Poor," reinforcing what we see in Smit's engraving: the devastating effects of cattle disease on farmers whose animals were infected. Once infection broke out among their cattle, eighteenth-century farmers could expect sometimes entire herds to succumb—even without preventative slaughter—within a few weeks, if not days; government compensation at best enabled the farmer to restock only half of their herds. Farriers, cow-leeches, and those dependent on the industry were equally affected, as were London's poor. A rising population had been driving up food prices at the same time that an increasing number of England's working population had been removed from agricultural labor. By 1750, as Raj Patel and Jason Moore argue, England's role as the "bread-basket of Europe" (2018, 142) reached a "tipping point," most of its population driven off the land and into cities. Indeed, the rapid increase of enclosure acts between 1760 and 1790—six times as many as in the previous three decades—itself may have been a response to epidemic realities of cattle plague (Patel and Moore 2018, 143). Farmers and the poor, then, overwhelmed by no-win decisions and threatened by starvation, felt cattle plague more immediately and more intensely than did large landowners, who still received their rents. In fact, landowners often demanded the government compensation payments, intended for farmers who had lost cattle to cattle disease, so they could offset the rent arrears from their tenants.

This dire situation was exacerbated (as with bubonic and other human plagues) by unending and usually false advertisements for cures, by flagging confidence in the effectiveness of cull and slaughter policies, and by genuine confusion about how best to respond to a disease so poorly understood. The *Philosophical Transactions* of 1745 includes a November paper entitled "Some Account of the Distemper raging among the Cow-kind in the neighborhood of London, together with some Remedies proposed for their Recovery" by Cromwell Mortimer, secretary of the Royal Society, along with two follow-ups (Mortimer 1745b, Mortimer 1746).[2]

[2] In addition to Mortimer's papers in the *Philosophical Transactions of the Royal Society* see Lobb (1745, 382–83); and, for a list of related works, Mullet (1946: 144–65).

Mortimer begins by recommending the policies of Thomas Bates, recently advocated by Theophilus Lobb, but offers a perspective from the "Cowkeepers" who tell him that a cow may appear to be well, and "feed heartily over night" but that in "twelve Hours time" they will neither eat or drink; the next day they "hang down their Heads" (1745a, 533). The third day they purge, "groan much, and seem to be in great Pain." Cattle left "out in the cold" (533–34) seldom live beyond three days; those in warm stalls might last for seven. "The concern the cow-keepers are under for the loss of their substance," Mortimer writes in his next letter, "the various methods offered to them, and their want of judgment either to chuse the most rational, or their want of accuracy in making experiments, and following directions, is quite discouraging….indeed, several own to me, they are quite bewildered, not knowing which way to turn themselves, or whose advice to follow, what one says being quite contrary to the directions given by another" (1745b, 552). Mortimer's description of the farmers' confusion mirrors what Kurth and Pikhala have described as practical anxiety about ecological matters, the experience of uncertainty about the right thing to do in the face of ecological threats and challenges (2022). Today, we are probably more accustomed to thinking of practical eco-anxiety in relation to climate change: "should I recycle?" "should I boycott"? "should I protest?" For eighteenth-century farmers whose cattle may or may not be showing signs of suffering, the questions are even more immediately thanatonic: "do I kill"? "do I treat?" "do I report?" "do I (illegally) sell?" Given the probability of complete or partial herd mortality, rapidly changing government policies, and the many ineffective medical treatments on offer, Mortimer's claim that the farmers are "bewildered," or lost in a pathless place ("not knowing which way to turn themselves"), captures the practical eco-anxiety generated by mass animal die-offs.

The indecision and bewilderment among "Cowkeepers" that Mortimer describes resonates with the dilemma facing physicians, writers, and their readers: efforts to seek scientific explanations for outbreaks by looking at authoritative texts set against the tendency to fall back, as in *De Mortibus Boum*, on prayer and penitence. The touchstone for many literate Englishmen and women in the seventeenth and eighteenth centuries remained Virgil's *Georgics*. Virgil's account of a mass mortality event in the *Georgics* offers one of the most detailed descriptions of cattle plague. As Frans De Bruyn has argued, many eighteenth-century translators approached Virgil as a "scientific" writer, and they were "predisposed to make strong cognitive claims for the poem, not simply as a didactic and instructional document but as a text that conveyed systematic technical and scientific knowledge on matters agricultural" (de Bruyn 2005, 150).[3] In the eighteenth century, Virgil's plague description helped ground a tradition that includes not only major literary figures, such as John Dryden and Abraham Cowley, but a host of lesser-known Virgil translators and adapters like William Benson, John Martyn, and James Hamilton. Reading Virgil in the original or in translation may have helped to shape perceptions of cattle plague, perhaps as much as contemporary agricultural treatises.

John Dryden's influential 1697 translation of the *Georgics* highlights Virgil's "systematic technical and scientific knowledge" about cattle and grain economies, including a sensitivity to the effects of seasonal variability or disruption on livestock. Dryden includes a powerful warning about the devastating effects of winter on herds and flocks:

> On Winter Seas we fewer Storms behold,
> Than foul Diseases that infect the Fold.
> Nor do these ills, on single Bodies prey;
> But oft'ner bring the Nation to decay;
> And sweep the present Stock, and future Hope away. (233; Georgic III, 5: ll. 711–715).

Dryden makes clear the stakes in outbreaks of cattle plague, partly because of their scale. Because rinderpest afflicts the "Nation" rather than "single Bodies," countries that depend on agriculture, rather than on trade (like Shakespeare's Venice), will "decay" with the death of their livestock. In ways that recall cattle plague in *De Mortibus Boum*, both the "present Stock" and the "future Hope," their offspring, will succumb to the same "foul" disease. Following this grim stanza are 130 gory lines about the "Strange" deaths of sacrificial oxen, calves, swine, dogs, horses, buffalo, wolves, fish, snakes, and birds, as well as an especially affecting version of the bovine elegy featuring a dying ox. The poem conveys the translator's despair, as well as Virgil's, about the possibility of medical intervention:

> Besides, to change their Pasture 'tis in vain:
> Or trust to Physic; Physic is their Bane.

[3] On Dryden's translations, see Caldwell (2000) and Caldwell (2008).

> The learned Leaches in despair depart:
> And shake their Heads, desponding of their Art. (236, 5: ll. 816–820)

Because Dryden is translating a classical, pre-Christian poem, he bypasses an opportunity to frame cattle plague as an instrument of God's judgment. The "learned Leeches," instead, like the dying livestock, exist in a world where the operations of nature seem irrevocable, beyond human and even divine intervention. Both Virgil and Dryden ascribe murrain to Tisiphone, one of the three Furies, who "treads the round," then strikes "an Universal Blow": "To Death at once whole Herds of Cattle go:/ Sheep, Oxen, Horses fall: and, heap'd on high,/ The diff'ring Species in Confusion lie" (ll. 829–31). Determined by a relentless fate, cattle plague must be endured rather than prayed away. Book Three of Dryden's translation ends with a disease mitigation policy in keeping with best practices still relevant 1600 years after Virgil wrote the *Georgics*, with mass burial: "the way they found,/ To lodge their loathsome Carrion underground" (ll. 831–32). Animals' hides are "useless," and the flesh irredeemably "tainted"; even fleece shorn from dead sheep crawls with lice that produce "Red Blisters," "flaming Carbuncles," and "clammy Dews" (ll. 840–842). While the lice may recall buprestis or other noxious insects, Dryden broadens the imagery to something approaching utter destruction: "'Til the slow creeping Evil eats his way/ Consumes the parching Limbs; and makes the Life his prey" (844–45). As a "slow creeping Evil," then, cattle plague appears both as vermicular infestation and as an apex predator that "eats" and "Consumes" not only the individual lives of animals and humans, but "the Life" of the biopolitical order itself.

But in addition to desperate cures, inconsistent policies, and poetic fatalism, England's mid-century outbreaks of endemic livestock disease also generated more than their share of hymns and religious reflections. The official prayer for the nation's herds, composed by the Archbishop of Canterbury in 1748, was, as John Hardwick notes, "prescribed for daily use" throughout the Church of England for "an extraordinarily long time," (2024, 158) until 1759. Hardwick points to a tension or awkwardness in his excellent summary of the Anglican prayers. Even though cattle had a special religious meaning for Christians—Jesus, after all, was born in a manger—prayers for cattle raised difficult questions, including why "God would punish innocent animals for human sins" (158). Dissenters, by contrast, were more comfortable with taking up the suffering and death of plague-stricken animals as part of religious thought. Hardwick mentions a sermon by Samuel King, who represents cattle as being "close to God," their "suffering groans…a means by which God spoke to human communities," especially to "those in need of repentance and reform" (159). Typical in this regard are the works of dissenting Reverend Philip Doddridge (1702–1751), who lived through two major rinderpest events. Included among his more than sixty hymns is "The Hand of the Lord upon the Cattle," based on Exodus 9.3: "Behold, the hand of the Lord *is* upon thy cattle, which is in the field, upon the horse, upon the horses, upon the asses, upon the camels, upon the oxen, and upon the sheep: *there shall be* a very grievous murrain" (Doddridge 1755, 5). This posthumously published hymn contains three familiar features: detailed descriptions of dying cattle, an insistence on their innocence, and a call for humans, who brought down the scourge, to repent their sins. The second stanza begins with a plea to God to "hear" the moaning Cattle as they succumb to the plague, and the third ends by framing the disease of "harmless" animals as a sign of human sin:

> O look from thine exalted Throne,
> And hear our panting Cattle moan;
> Prone o'er th' untasted Food they lye,
> Groan out their Agonies, and dye.
> What have these harmless Creatures done
> To draw this sore Chastisement down?
> 'Tis human Guilt for Vengeance calls,
> And heavy on the Herds it falls. (Doddridge 1755, 5)

These lines reaffirm familiar religious interpretations of livestock disease. Doddridge's fourth stanza, moreover, in keeping with the temporality and continuity of the plagues visited on the Egyptians, looks toward the sixth plague and consequently to the possibility of zoonotic transmission:

> From them to us the Stroke might pass,
> And mow down Thousands of our Race:
> Till Desolation reign'd around,
> Our Cities void, untill'd our Ground. (Doddridge 1755, 5)

By "Stroke" Doddridge means the disease sent by God that could "pass" from animal to humans. Early modern writers and artists intuited connections between dying cattle and dying humans in their depictions of the plague, as I discussed in Chap. 1; Doddridge's hymn suggests that scientific debates about rinderpest could still be accommodated within a familiar agrotheology. The hymn ends, therefore, with a hopeful plea, or fantasy, that this visitation may be preventative, a warning that might "melt our Hearts to seek [God's] Face"; more precisely, the dead cattle appear as signs of God's merciful guidance: "Blest Fruit of thy correcting Rod/ To lose our Beasts, and find our GOD" (5). Doddridge transmutes the despair and economic ruin depicted in Smit's print into traditional homiletic, an appeal to repent.

Cattle plague as blessed warning also appears in James Hervey's 1746 *Meditations and Contemplations*, which went through fourteen editions in as many years. While Hervey, who regarded himself as a "moderate Calvinist," emphasizes the innocence of the beasts, he links the ongoing epizootic to the failed Jacobite rebellion of 1745.[4] The rebellion has been suppressed—"the sword of civil discord" returned "into its sheath"—but the nation, he claims, has not learned to forego its evil ways. Because the English have not "become a renewed people" devoted to a dying "Savior," the innocent cattle must suffer. "No wantoness or sloth has vitiated the blood of these laborious, temperate creatures," Hervey writes in *Contemplations on the Night*:

> They have contracted no disease from unseasonable indulgences and inordinate revellings... Neither care disturbs their sleep nor passion inflames their breast. Whence, then, are they visited with such terrible disorders, as no prudence can prevent, nor any medicines heal? (1808, 2: 214)

Although Hervey's ostensible subject in this passage is the night sky as evidence of providential design, the "disorders" described in morbid detail mimic eighteenth-century prayers, bovine elegies, and reports from physicians: "What mean those peals of sobs which burst from the expiring cattle?" he asks, "What mean those melancholy moans, where the lusty droves were meant to low?" (1808, 2: 214) Hervey, like Doddridge, renders the suffering of these animals in recognizably human ways—in sobs, in melancholy moans—to forge an affective link between animals and humans that then can be wrested into an acknowledgment of collective human sin. "Surely these calamities are the weapons of Divine displeasure, and manifest chastisements of an evil generation," he writes, but they are also a

[4] On fear in Hervey's poetry and sermons, see Parisot (2015: 121–35).

warning: "Surely God," he claims, "the 'God to whom vengeance belongeth,' has still a controversy with our sinful land. And who can tell where the visitations will end?" (2: 215) Like Doddridge, Hervey holds open the possibility of contagious disease passing from cattle to humans, who bear the "Guilt" of God's "manifest chastisements." Dying cattle, then, function paradoxically as real, suffering animals and as occasions for human spiritual metamorphosis. Only because cattle are feeling and suffering beings whose "moans" and "sobs" bring them within the compass of human sentiment can Hervey and Doddridge provoke guilt and repentance in "an evil generation." Doddridge's hymn and Hervey's meditation define the affective contours of the bovine elegy.

The most famous—or infamous—literary meditation on expiring cattle, however, belongs to William Dodd (1729–1777), an Anglican clergyman and sometimes literati whose expenses exceeded the fruits of his preferments. Entitled "Diggon Davy's resolution on the death of his last cow," it was his first publication, appearing in 1747. Every reference to this poem, including Dodd's own, takes pains to mention the occasion of its writing "in order to convince a friend, that the distemper which then prevailed amongst the horned cattle, had been described by Virgil."[5] Although Dodd was a clergyman, given his devotion to Virgil, "Diggon Davy" takes a different tack on cattle plague than many of the more overtly religious texts, like Doddridge's and Hervey's. Dodd reproduces the ecological fatalism that creeps into many of the translations of Virgil in the eighteenth century, including Dryden's. Notwithstanding Dodd's desire to link his poem to the *Georgics*, apparent in his annotations, "Diggon Davy" nevertheless has as much in common with *De Mortibus Boum* and sentimental literature as it does with Virgil.

Dodd's pastoral differs from the *Georgics* in focusing on cows alone and features two shepherds, Diggon and Colin, meeting in the contagious fields. Diggon laments that this new cattle plague, "where every gale contains the seeds of death," has taken both Mully and Susan. Having tried all the recommended cures to no avail—"Med'cines I gave, like poison med'cines flew" (261)—he describes in agonizing detail Susan's death:

> Dejected first she hung her drooping head,
> Refus'd her meat, and from her pasture fled;

[5] See the anonymous biography, *An authentick account of the late unfortunate Doctor William Dodd*, 1777.

Then dull and languid seem'd her plaintive eye
Her breath grew noisome, and her udder dry…
Scorch'd with perpetual thirst, short sighs she drew;
Furr'd was her tongue, and to her mouth it grew:
Her burning nostrils putrid rheums distill'd,
And death's strong agonies her bowels fill'd;
Each limb contracted, and a groan each breath,
Lost ease I wish'd her, and it came in death:
Cast out, infected, and abhorr'd by all;
See how the useful, and the beauteous fall!
Not eve'n her skin—when living, sleek and red,
Can aught avail me, Colin, now she's dead. (262–63)

Susan's symptoms depart little from those described by writers going back to Topsell and Markham: mouth lesions ("furr'd tongue"), discharge from the nose ("her nostrils putrid rheums distill'd"), diarrhea ("death's strong agonies her bowles fill'd"), and dehydration, ultimately leading to death. Susan also experiences emotional responses to her illness; she is "Dejected," "dull," "and languid," her groans suggesting not only physical pain but a consciousness of what is happening to her. Diggon grieves Susan's death, even as he calculates his financial loss at being unable to sell her hide.

A mash-up of Virgil and sentimental literature, "Diggon Davy" is affectively unstable. Although, as, in different ways, Keith Thomas, Laura Brown, and Tobias Menely have demonstrated, certain animals—lapdogs, primates, singing birds, among them—had by mid-century entered the affective community of "sensibility" writing, dying cows never quite made the affective grade.[6] Diggon's details about Susan's "beauteous" skin, then, render the favorite cow a near-erotic object, and the poem a kind of bovine snuff porn. Or, stripped of its epidemiological entanglements, "Diggon Davy" easily appears as an extended joke about the rustic sentimentality of Dodd's farmer lamenting the death and implied sexiness of his cow. Yet as the son of a clergyman from Bourne, in Lincolnshire, Dodd had grown up in English cattle country, an origin likely evident in his description of Susan's "skin—when living, sleek and red." The Lincoln

[6] See Thomas (1983); Brown (2017); Brown (2023); and Menely (2015). Nathaniel Wolloch argues that pet culture and the sensibility it engendered were selective, at best. See Wolloch (2006). On the affective connections to other animals, including cows, in the sixteenth and seventeenth centuries, see Fudge (2018).

Red of his birthplace is one of the oldest native breeds in England. When embedded in the trauma of cattle plague and bolstered by Dodd's conceptual framing in its georgic allusions to Virgil, the poem assumes a kind of affective pathos, one grounded in breed specificity and realism about futile efforts to manage a disease that remains "one of the most heavy calamities that can befall any European country" (Dossie 482) Anticipating how the absence of an interpretive frame could twist the poem into a satire, Dodd includes in most editions a note that the poem was written in 1747, when distemper "reined" among the "horned cattle."

Dodd's nervousness about how literari and literary critics would receive his bovine elegy is well founded. Noting that there had been a "terrible disease among the cattle" from which his "parish had suffered greatly," Laurence Sterne, for example, recounts bits of a "spiritual song" from a "parochial bard" delivered from the pulpit; "not only the murrain itself, but the sufferers by the calamity," he writes to a friend, "were vociferated through the aisles in all the pomp and devotion of rustic psalmody" (Sterne 1788, 62–63). He repeats the last stanza in a letter:

> Here's Jemmy How has lost a cow
> And so has Johnny Bland;
> Therefore we'll put our trust in God
> And not in any other man.

Tongue in cheek, Sterne quips that this verse "rather unhinged my devotion, but it seemed to rivet that of the congregation, and therefore I have no right to complain" (63). Sterne recoils in a well-mannered way both from the performance of the "spiritual song," its "pomp and devotion," and apparently from the subject—murrain, dying cows, desolated farmers. His delicate jibes at the agrarian congregation riveted by a "rustic psalmody," however, have moral and economic consequences for Jemmy How and Johnny Bland. The bovine elegy opens a window to a material history of disease to which all quadrupeds are vulnerable; some people are more vulnerable than others; and poor people are most vulnerable of all. The aesthetic quality of a poem like "Diggon Davy" may be debatable for an Anglican cleric, a failed farmer, and late-life novelist like Sterne, but its implications for his parishioners are not.

Dodd returned to the subject of cattle plague in a second pastoral poem, "The Good Old Woman," who is praised for bringing "relief/ To beds of sickness, and the house of grief." Lucy, the narrator, specifies the source of that "grief," the loss of sheep and cattle:

> When late the rot consum'd our flocks around.
> When just before the murrain spread the ground
> With carcases of cattle—strangely dead!
> And every farmer hung his drooping head:
> Remember, how from house to house she went,
> Consoling all, and minist'ring content:
> That—to the stroke of Providence resign'd,
> A murmerer 'mongst us it was hard to find! (223)

Providing economic, emotional, and spiritual comfort to stricken farmers (who, like the dying cattle, are characterized by a "drooping head"), Dodd suggests, is necessary to social stability in a time of crisis. "The Good Old Woman" offers a political counterpart to Sterne's snickering at the amateurish poem about the effects of cattle plague on the Jemmys and Johnnys of the parish. The poor in Dodd's poem are asked to resign themselves to "the stroke of Providence," to remain "content" and quiet, literally without a murmur, despite having been devastated financially. Without the Virgilian notes that contextualize cattle plague in "Diggon Davy," Dodd's Old Woman can give voice to long-standing Christian admonitions to patience in the face of trials. Her "minist'ring content" functions to deflect growing rural resentment about the ineptitude and overreach of the government's plague mitigation efforts.

To return to Ritvo's point about eighteenth-century references to cattle plague seeming both ephemeral and comparatively sparse, I have argued that because the epizootics have differential effects on different populations, mostly affecting economically vulnerable rural farmers and villagers, we need to look closely at the ways cattle plague is buried in a wide variety of texts—hymns, prayers, topical poetry—written *during* or soon after the outbreaks, rather than years later when the plagues are recollected in tranquility or half-forgotten. Oliver Goldsmith appears far more sympathetic to the farmers than does Laurence Sterne. In the 1770s, after yet another outbreak, Goldsmith describes the dire plight of the poor in his *History of the Earth and Animated Nature.* In "Quadrepedes of the Cow Kind," he calls the cow—as distinct from sheep or the horse, which is "an animal belonging to the rich"—"the poor man's pride, his riches, and his support" (1774, 3: 8). There are "many of our peasantry that have no other possession but a cow," he continues, even though they are but "nominal possessors" of the advantages it offers.

> Its flesh they cannot pretend to taste, since then their whole riches are at once destroyed; its calf they are obliged to fatten for sale, since veal is a delicacy they could not make any pretensions to; its very milk is wrought into butter and cheese for the tables of their masters; while they have no share even in their own possession, but the choice of their market. (3: 8)

Goldsmith offers here a significant critique of how the "Cow Kind" are commodified, distinguishing them from horses both by the labor they perform and by the costs the latter demand.[7] The poor fare better in Germany, Poland, and Switzerland, Goldsmith maintains, where the peasant keeps two or three cows "not for the benefit of his master, but for himself" (3: 9). Even the most impoverished citizens of these nations have at least one cow killed for their table, salted and "hung up" as a mark of hospitality, as an "elegant piece of furniture which, though seldom touched," at least "argues the possessors's elegance and ease," and often makes him "better contented with hunger" (3: 9). But "for some years past," he continues, it is very different "in this country, where our lower rustics at least are utterly unable to purchase meat any part of the year, and by them even butter is considered as an article of extravagance" (3: 9). One of these "lower rustics," obviously, functions as the persona of "Diggon Davy" and as the subject of "The Good Old Woman," comforting the "lower rustics" around her. And the yawning economic gap between such people and wealthy or even middle-class Englishmen explains why Goldsmith includes the following remark in his natural history of the cow: "I cannot bear to hear the rich crying out for liberty," he writes, "while they thus starve their fellow creatures, and feed them up with an imaginary good, while they monopolize the real benefits of nature" (3: 8). The cow, a "real benefit of nature," has been swallowed up by ongoing political disputes between Whigs—"crying out for liberty," but often supporting the slave trade, imperial expansion, industrialization, and expensive overseas wars designed to secure trade routes and trading factories in Asia—and Tories, wedded, at least in theory, to a traditional

[7] On Goldsmith's socioeconomic critiques of rural life, see Griffin (2013); Mason (2014: 21–39); and Van Renen (2023: 467–75). On the significance of horses in transnational elite cultures, see Landry (2009), and Landry (2011: 11–30).

vision of the English countryside, social stability, and aristocratic privileges. Goldsmith's critique of class privilege does not quite rise to the level of revolutionary fervor. But appearing in a section of his natural history devoted to "Quadrapedes of the Cow Kind," it exposes the hypocrisy of political movements that cannot or will not acknowledge the interdependencies between farmers and dying cows in an increasingly distempered natural world.[8]

Dossie's Cold Calculations: Eco-anxiety in the 1770s

Goldsmith's sarcastic line, "crying out for liberty," gestures to the ongoing turmoil in England's domestic and colonial politics, not only the rebellion brewing in the American colonies, but the conflicts between George III, who succeeded his grandfather in 1760, and Parliament. During the new king's first ten years, administrations changed seven times. By the time George III opened Parliament in January 1770, he was being petitioned by several counties and bodies for its dissolution and faced demands for the reform of election law. As the *Annual Register* describes this opening, "the nation had been in a great ferment during the whole summer—the like had scarcely been ever remembered" (1785, 58), in part because Parliament refused to seat the dissenter John Wilkes, publisher of the ostensibly seditious paper *North Briton*; although Wilkes had fled to France, in 1768 he nonetheless was elected MP for Middlesex.[9] Widely perceived as a martyr for liberty, Wilkes was championed by A Society for the Supporters of the Bill of Rights, founded in his name. "The minds of all men were occupied on the one side and the other with these considerations," reports the *Annual Register*, "and great expectations were formed concerning the manner in which these great points would be handled in the speech of January 9th, from the throne" (59). Instead of addressing "the great domestic movements" having to with the Middlesex election, however, the King "began, by taking notice of a distemper that had broke out among the horned cattle; touched some topics concerning foreign affairs, and the distractions of America, and concluded with the

[8] See Valenze (2006, 145–77 and 260–276); and Mitchell (2007).

[9] On Wilkes and the controversies around the *North Briton*, see Peter D. G. Thomas (1996, 70–89).

usual recommendation to unanimity" in the face of cattle plague (59). "I thought it absolutely necessary," the King declared,

> with the advice of my privy council, to give immediate directions for every step to be taken that appeared most capable of checking the instant danger of the spreading of the infection, until I could have an opportunity of consulting my parliament upon some more permanent measures for securing us against so great a calamity: And to your immediate and serious consideration I earnestly recommend this very important subject. (244)[10]

Despite the severity of the outbreak, many perceived the plague-centered speech as a distraction from parliamentary politics. Responses from periodicals were widely dismissive, even shocked that cattle distemper trumped electoral rights in the sovereign's priorities. Again, according to the *Register*:

> The public were much suprized at the silence concerning the petitions, and at the solemn mention of the horned cattle, which filled the place of that important business. It became even a subject of too general ridicule, especially as the existence of the distemper, or at least the extent or danger, did not dispose the people to more serious thoughts. (59)

Many years later, William Massey's *A History of England during the Reign of George III* echoes this view: "Never was a King's speech received with such an ebullition of ridicule and contempt" (1865, 1: 311). Political troubles at home and abroad, for most observers, should have eclipsed the significance of this third eighteenth-century outbreak of cattle plague.

Tensions between political concerns and public health often characterizes governmental responses to disease, as we know all too well in the twenty-first century. In this context, I find it fascinating that shortly after the appearance of Edmund Burke's *Thoughts on the Cause of the Present Discontents* (1770), Robert Dossie (who sometimes wrote under the pseudonym Agricola) published his second volume of *Memoirs of Agriculture, and other Œconomical Arts* which—in addition to introducing rhubarb, a new species of potato, and instructions for making bread—treated the cattle contagion as seriously as George III did in opening Parliament, though without having to dodge issues of electoral reform. While Dossie, to us, is a far less familiar name than Burke, to his

[10] *Annual Register for 1770*, State Papers, King's Speech, 9 January 1770.

contemporaries, like Samuel Johnson, he seemed an exemplar of useful knowledge, someone dedicated to linking the arts and sciences to commercial as well as technological progress. Long before he wrote *Memoirs of Agriculture* (which was in George III's library), Dossie had gained a significant reputation across Europe; his *Handmaid to the Arts* (1758) had explained the principles of color, design, and technique essential to material arts such as enameling (Kurzer 2004: 65–88). As a prominent member of the Society for Encouragement of Arts, Manufactures and Commerce, Dossie took seriously its mission: to cultivate experimental research, to collect information, and to transmit it to the public (Gibbs 1951, 145–172). In contrast to the husbandry manuals of the previous centuries, typically organized into entries of a few sentences or paragraphs, Dossie devotes over 120 pages of *Memoirs of Agriculture* to "Murrain, or Pestilential Disease of Neat Cattle." He apologizes for, but defends, the length of this essay, justifying his ambitious effort to treat the rinderpest outbreak as a social, cultural, and economic calamity worth serious and sustained attention. "Nothing of this kind, so perfect as to be of any practical use, has been hitherto given to the public in any language" (368), he contends. His now under-read essay stakes a claim to offer a workable policy for tackling cattle plague that, he argues, is both scientifically valid and economically viable.

Insisting on the importance of distinguishing among the diseases that afflict cattle, Dossie advocates returning to the old name of "murrain" for the disease "raging at times in most countries of Europe; and carrying such destruction wherever it comes that it may be truly deemed a pestilence of the cattle" (364–65). Having noted the King's recent speech (366n), he advocates for a national effort, "some proper plan," for the "prevention and cure" of murrain. Although he acknowledges that many "academic bodies" have been called on by the government to "deliver their opinions on" the current outbreak, in his mind their recommendations are based less on experimental observation than on habitual practice, and therefore have resulted in little of "practical utility" (368). Drawing on experiments recently conducted in the Netherlands, he proposes a "new" approach based on a "new principle": that murrain is neither typically contagious nor primarily local but seasonal and a matter of the cattle's vulnerability to disease. Although Dossie may exaggerate the novelty of his approach, he presents it as an improvement over cull and bury policies, which, he asserts, have been both socially divisive and economically impractical.

His treatise focuses on two interrelated aspects of animals' vulnerability: the role of climate in infection and the cost of trying to cure sick animals. Although, as we have seen, poets from Virgil to Thomson, not to mention authors of husbandry manuals, suggest that cattle disease is seasonal or that it flourishes under certain climatic conditions, Dossie offers scientific evidence, drawn from British history as well as from contemporary Dutch experiments, that the murrain is "an epidemical disease, though contagious" that arises only "when certain unfavorable circumstances of season have created a predisposition in the cattle to receive the infection; and thence rendered them temporarily susceptible of it" (399). Rather than look for specific agents of transmission—like insects—he identifies environmental factors, individually or in combination, that make cattle prone to "epidemical disease": "moist air, replete with putrid vapours," "a long continuance of easterly winds," "severe cold," and "repeated alternations of heat and cold in the weather" (376). All these factors affect harvests and consequently food supplies. The protracted outbreak in the Netherlands, he argues, can be attributed to "a longer series than common of unfavorable seasons conspiring with the great relaxation natural to the cattle in so damp a country"; similar conditions obtained in "every part of Europe" after 1711, a period, as we saw in the last chapter, of widespread epizootics "when the season had been so inclement the year before, as to destroy a great part of the sheep in England; and again in 1741… as a very intense frost, which lasted from December to April" (376). The conditions that led to earlier epizootics in England, he suggests, can always return and start the deadly cycle over again. In 1741, for example, the "rigour of cold, and scarcity of fodder . . . reduced the cattle in general to a debilitated state: which was still aggravated by the almost constant easterly winds that blew the summer and autumn following" (376).[11] Although "more clement weather" helped to mitigate cattle disease later in the decade, murrain returned in various places and times. Recently, he claims, the "irregularities" of the seasons, "the great alternations of heat and cold," "and the frequency of easterly winds" have conspired to weaken "both vegetables and animals," rendering "the cattle peculiarly susceptible of this infection, as well as mankind of those contagious distempers to which they are subject" (365n).

[11]The cold condition in the early 1740s resulted, in part, from aerosols spewed into the atmosphere by volcanic eruptions in the Far East. See David MacCallum (2019); Wood (2014).

Although Dossie links animal and human disease in this note, he is adamant that climate and the constitutions of individual bodies are the driving factors in the spread of epidemics.

Dossie's claims about animals' vulnerability to ecological factors anticipate, in many ways, those of some contemporary environmental historians. Drawing on scholars who have argued that the Justinian plague was "triggered by, or associated with climatic anomalies," Timothy Newfield argues convincingly for a "causal connection" between cattle plagues and climate in the Early Middle Ages, but one "dependent on intermediary factors" (2015, 97) such as famine. Sam White, similarly, makes a broader case for the relationship between climate change and mass mortality events. He argues that climate contributes to famine, and famine makes populations vulnerable to diseases, whether contagious or not. From this perspective, the Little Ice Age's long wet summers and colder winters had cascading effects (White 2011). Without oxen, the plough falls idle; without grain, both humans and animals weaken from hunger; weak animals, both human and nonhuman, are more susceptible to plague. In the Ottoman territories, a series of freezing winters in the 1590s coincided with the worst drought in six centuries.[12] The cold and drought destroyed harvests and, White argues, "left livestock exposed and starving, leading to a major epizootic that decimated sheep and cattle over much of Anatolia, the Crimea, and the Balkans" (White 2010, 559). "Rather than simply counting plague outbreaks," White advises, "we need to look more closely at factors that mitigated or aggravated exposure and vulnerability to infection, such as climate, nutrition, migration, and economic and political stability" (2010, 558). Environmental scholars like Newfield and White are not arguing for deterministic causal connections—bad weather brings disease—but exploring the implications that, in Newfield's words, the "probability" of links among climate phenomena, famine, and mass animal die-offs "is high" (117).

Dossie's thesis about the susceptibility of cattle to seasonal irregularities, though, cannot be straitjacketed into readings of contemporary literary texts or viewed simply as anticipating our own ecological concerns. *Memoirs of Agriculture, and other Œconomical Arts* emerges from and responds to a charged political environment and seeks to counter government policies, in place since the 1711 epizootic, of culling diseased

[12] Sam White, "Rethinking Disease in Ottoman," *International Journal of Middle East Studies* 42, 4 (2010), 559.

animals. Dossie agrees with culling programs for the sake of "national security" when the disease is "confined to one spot only" (454–455n), but widespread epidemics—as in the Netherlands, and in past visitations—make such a scheme impractical, even destructive. When murrain has "spread over a large extent," destroying cattle would lead to "scarcity" and therefore "would cooperate with the disease itself" (455n). In ways that seem to dovetail with contemporary breed improvement programs, he urges abandoning early plague mitigation policies inherited from Ramazzini, Lancisi, and Bates (see Chap. 4). Instead, he emphasizes the importance of cultivating "strength"—almost a synonym for wellness—in animals. Drawing on "a very extensive field of observation," he insists that "both mankind and brutes are liable to the attacks of most contagious disorders in proportion to their defect of strength" (379). Culling, in this respect, becomes a last-ditch strategy for weakened animals in times of climatic stress. Because the health of the body politic depends on the health of cattle and their human keepers, Dossie advocates a set of policies to dampen the spread of infectious disease.

This turn to preventative health and wellness allows him to dismiss traditional attempts at curing murrain through mundification (cleansing), bleeding, blisters, rowels, caustics, purging, antiseptics, alexiphramics (antidotes to poisons), emollients, and sedatives. Many of these remedies were based on the assumption that murrain is an "inflammatory" disease, like smallpox or the plague. Layard, among others, assumed that this was the case. But Dossie systematically rejects this view. Such faulty medical regimes have been constructed, he claims, on the "erroneous foundation" of an "analogy" between smallpox and murrain; he reasons there cannot be any "affinity" among smallpox, plague, and murrain, because the inoculation of beasts neither "hinder[s] their receiving the infection again" nor prevents them from dying of the disease (394, 395n). Moreover, smallpox symptoms include both fevers and eruptions of "morbid matter," which sometimes presage individuals' recoveries; in murrain, by contrast, similar eruptions sometimes are "wholly wanting," even when the beasts recover, and therefore are not, he reasons, "essential to the disease" (414n). In Dossie's view, these traditional treatments are actively counterproductive. They "disturb" the "animal œconomy," "weakening the beasts" and rendering them "more subject to the malignant action of the contagion" (412). In brief, ineffective efforts to cure diseased cattle are both epidemiologically dubious and economically dangerous.

Instead, Dossie advocates for medicines that invigorate and strengthen animals, notably Peruvian Bark (chinoa bark, Jesuit's bark), which the physician James Lind had recently called "the most powerful and Strengthener and Restorative of enfeebled, languid Constitutions, and the only Specific yet known for the malignant Diseases" (Lind 1763, 133) prevalent in tropical climates. Known for its use in so-called tropical medicine against malaria and typhus, or "ship's fever," Peruvian bark was also being tested by this time on patients with catalepsy, epilepsy, and other diseases in the Royal Infirmary in Edinburgh (formerly known as Hospital for the Sick Poor) and elsewhere (Maehle 2013, 150–155). Despite his belief that Peruvian bark could fortify cattle against disease, any public health program, Dossie admits, must be "practicable, with a moderate share of expense and trouble; or it will never be put in practice, by the proprietors of the cattle" (422). Even the most "able" of the physicians, he asserts, including Layard, need to recognize that "an effectual plan for the saving any material number of the cattle" must be financially viable. The cure must allow the farmer to make a profit on the surviving animal; if the cure is too expensive, it makes more sense "to abandon [cattle] to the effects of this disease" (423). The "great obstacle"—the *only* obstacle—in prescribing Peruvian bark in sufficient qualities is its "high price" (447). While it *could* be used preventatively, Dossie argues that such a regime would be uneconomical. "To put a larger herd of cattle under a medicinal regimen, and continue it so for a long time, would most obviously be attending with a certain great loss, for the precarious chance of avoiding another loss, that, at worst, could not be equal to it" (406–07). Put simply, to use Peruvian bark as a preventative would cost more than the value of the herd. Instead, Dossie recommends several cheap and available substitutes (tormental root, a cordial made of caraway seed, fermented liquors, chalk in their feed) (452). Admitting that no regime can "avail in every instance" (452), he suggests that if enough cattle survive to justify "the expense of the treatment," confounded and financially strapped cattle owners will be inclined to try this regime, and the "public" will "reap great advantage" (452, 454). Dossie's cost-benefit analysis yokes a detailed medical critique of treatments for cattle disease to a pounds-and-pence view of how preventative regimes might actually work. Rather than an argument, like Goldsmith's, about the value of the cows to the poor and the indifference of the "rich," Dossie subsumes affective concerns for suffering animals and struggling farmers into a conceptual spreadsheet for the nation as a whole—the "public" who will benefit from fewer market disruptions and cheaper meat.[13]

I emphasize Dossie's discussion of Peruvian bark and its substitutes to foreground two related issues, both relevant to what we would now call bioinsecurity: economic calculations and affective relations between humans and animals. First, Dossie's necropolitical spreadsheet offers a measure of the distance between England's eighteenth-century livestock industry and the best practices of the early modern period, when Leonard Mascall was warning against increasing herd sizes for the same of profit alone: "As great a praise to him that saves,/ As he that can increase" (Mascall 1587, av). While no less committed to curing cattle than Mascall, Dossie's ideal farmer metes out life and death according to medical and economic algorithms. Based on mortality rates in the Netherlands, medicine can at best save only one in two animals. Most proposed methods of cure, including his own Peruvian bark, would range from £5 to £10 an animal, a prohibitive expense for most owners, especially since when the murrain "last raged" in England, a certifiably diseased cow near London "was deemed" to be worth sixteen pounds, of which the farmer would get half (453n). In some cases, the cure costs more than the expected profit; in others, farmers would find it in their "interests to submit to the present loss," and take the government disbursement (424n). Dossie's bargain medical regime, in contrast—although not as effective as Peruvian bark—would amount to 32 shillings per beast. Even though only half of the animals would survive (if his experimental conclusions hold) that half would be enough to keep "up the national stock," and prevent the "scarcity from becoming greater." As significantly, because the price of cattle rises in times of plague, the owners of surviving cattle would find the "value" of their stock rising "very considerably" (453n).

The supposed advantage of Dossie's medical regime, then, is based less on the *real* value of cattle on an open market than on the policies of the sprawling government plague bureaucracy, including the compensation for animals that would ordinarily have to be culled. Oxen, bulls, cows, and calves are always-already perceived *both* as a collective financial entity expected to yield profit *and* as sick individuals whose real suffering could threaten the health of the herd, the national "stock," and thus the security of a nation. The herd itself, in other words, has become an abstract

[13] On the role of systems of calculation in the eighteenth century, see Markley (1999: 153–173), and Porter (2019).

value—a future profit that can be realized only if enough healthy animals can be brought to market. The individual medical attention that the farmer devotes to an animal, in this scenario, is largely a hedge against future losses; but the farmer can soon reach a tipping point where treatment "costs" more in terms of labor, time, and resources than can be justified on economic grounds. Cattle are locked inevitably, fatally, into an economic system in which the length and quality of their lives are sacrificed to a collective and politicized monetary abstraction.

Second, Dossie's calculations help make apparent, again, that cattle occupy a special place in Christian agrotheology, and consequently in the discourses of eighteenth-century economic thought, notably, Nathaniel Wolloch argues, (2006), in the works of Adam Smith. In the eighteenth-century georgic, affecting images of suffering beasts became a cornerstone of the discourse of a more-than-human sensibility. Tobias Menely has taught us to read such images of suffering animals as the basis of a "claim of ethical consideration" that implies a relation "between affective *communication* and interspecies *community*" (Menely 2006, 112). But, for livestock, as Menely would doubtless admit, images of suffering are nested within a complex set of connections. As Dossie's medical advice makes clear, affective relations and financial considerations are inseparable for animals in the food system. Even Diggon laments that he cannot sell Susan's hide. Unlike the dogs and cats of eighteenth-century pet culture—or even the hunted hares and foxes that became a rallying point for anti-cruelty polemics—cattle are always already overdetermined by the projected profits they can bring. These projections—we might even call them *fictions*—of future financial gain, nonetheless, are haunted by fears of catastrophic loss: an epizootic and subsequent cull, destroying herds.

The complete capture of cattle (and humans) in intertwined economic and medical regimes can be illustrated by looking at Francis Spilsbury's response to the Medicine Stamp Duty. Introduced by Lord John Cavendish in 1783, the duty at first taxed certain vendors for the medicines they sold: anyone who had served as apprentice to a surgeon, apothecary chemist, druggist, or military surgeon was exempt from paying the tax, as were those who had been licensed under the royal patent. Although the reasons for instituting this tax are "far from clear," in an era when "most serious diseases" (like murrain) could not be "cured, relieved, or prevented" by orthodox medical practices, the trade in so-called quack medicines, some of them actively dangerous, had proliferated; moreover, Britain's wars with America and others had left the treasury "seriously depleted," with a national debt of £234,000,000 (Stebbings 2014, 6). After the first version of the tax failed to raise sufficient revenues, the second, which William Pitt proposed two years later, yielded £12,000 the first year through one major change: it taxed the medicine rather than the vendor. Despite several exemptions, including one for "ordinary" medicines, the public outcry was fierce and immediate (Stebbings, 4). Opponents of the tax argued that medicines were necessities, not luxuries, and, under this heading, brought cattle and their diseases into the debate.

Francis Spilsbury, silversmith turned chemist, turned medical entrepreneur, and author of a 1775 treatise on curing gout, scurvy, leprosy, and the king's evil, entered the fray with a searing critique of Pitt's medicine tax, *The Power of Gold Displayed: in the Humane Proposal of the Right Hon. William Pitt, Chancellor of the Exchequer, to Bring Forward an Act to put His Majesty into the Disagreeable Situation of Signing a Decree, that no Sick or Lame person, or Diseased Cattle,...shall have a Medicine of Repute without Paying Tribute.* Arguing that the tax "places the Life of a human Being in competition with a Three-penny or Six-penny stamp," and, like a criminal warrant, "ends with an order for the execution of a fellow creature" (1785a, 3), Spilsbury links medicines required for cattle and human diseases; indeed, the title of his treatise claims that poor rural people—*not* those who can afford the tax—will suffer most in trying to treat their afflicted animals. "Is it not, ye guardians of the land," he asks, "a sore affliction to the owner of cattle, to hear his beast low with pain? Is that beast, or is an infant dying with disease, an object of taxation?" (3) In ways that evoke the groaning beasts of bovine elegies, but yoke them to helpless infants, Spilsbury accuses Pitt of taking advantage of human and animal distress. In a later version of this argument, addressed to booksellers who would be responsible for selling the stamp, Spilsbury accuses the monarch of breaking with tradition of caring for the health of his "own diseased subjects" (1785b, 6). Although former "Kings of Albion" delighted to act "the physician's part," this tax deprives both man and beast of "the general benefits of medicine," which Spilsbury describes as "Heaven's gift ... by providence ... designed to be as free for all nature's children as the air we breathe, or the water of the earth" (1785b, 6). Pitt's "brutal act" calls into questions distinctions between human and animal; man "talks of reformation, or more refined notions" but he quickly forgets the "dignity of his station" and, in the name of monetary self-interest, "devours his fellow creature," thereby raising the question—note the allusion to Rochester's

"Satire against Reason and Mankind"—of "which deserves the epithet of brute most, man or beast?" (1785b, 5)

As the patent holder for Spilsbury's Antiscorbutic Drops, which sold for five shillings, Spilsbury, Spilsbury's outrage, his objections to the tax, and his rhetoric of medicine as "Heaven's gift," must be taken with a grain of salt. The point I want to emphasize is that the language of sensibility that structures his treatise just as accurately could be called the language of vulnerability—specifically, vulnerability to epidemic diseases that affect humans and animals alike. Who can "avoid pity," Spilsbury asks at the beginning of an epic sentence, in seeing "even a dog in pain," and yet "officers of the crown" are empowered by the tax act to harass a "fellow creature, worried with the evil," his "soul chained to so vile a pestilential body," breathing vapors "poisonous" enough to "petrify" even "doctors"? (1785b, 5). Making full use of the idea that scrofulous ulcers leak pus that terrifies even medical professionals, Spilsbury contrasts this seemingly natural fear in the face of disease to the unfeeling, instrumental approach of Pitt and his medicine tax:

> Whilst from such diseased objects, and from diseased cattle, a Minister of State, with as much composure as a rat-catcher kills vermin, meditated an act of parliament which would pointedly militate against the welfare of the human and brute creation, loaded with insupportable infirmities, for he enacted that medicines of established reputation...should not be applied unless they gave a stipulated sum for a piece of paper. (1785b, 5)

In this extended metaphor, human and animal creation, especially cattle, are alike "loaded with insupportable infirmities." Rather than curing them, Pitt institutes taxes that amount to de facto extermination policies, like a "rat-catcher" killing "vermin." This metaphor has lost none of its power several hundred years later, as humans (and their animals) negotiate a medical industrial complex structured by profit that enforces its own cost-benefit analyses, increasingly, as in the United States, by private insurers rather than by patients or doctors. Whether applied to human or non-human patients, Spilsbury argues, placing profit over health is a dehumanizing impulse, a tax imposed by the wealthy on Goldsmith's poor farmers.

Cattle Plague and Bioinsecurity

In different ways, both Spilsbury and Dossie reveal the extent to which health, agriculture, government policies, and economics were linked inextricably by the late eighteenth century. Dossie's approach to cattle plague helped reinforce alternatives to the culling policies that had been on the books since the early eighteenth-century outbreaks. In this respect, his goals were aligned with those of an agricultural reform movement that appealed to nationalist and colonialist interests and increasingly captured the imagination of a wide swath of the population, including men like Samuel Johnson. Johnson knew Dossie and defended the marriage between commerce and husbandry in "Thoughts on Agriculture," published in 1756. Johnson argues in this text that readers "should look upon the English Farmer as the most useful member of society" and chastises both "Mankind" and "disposers of honorary awards" for having paid insufficient attention to "Agriculture" (1810a, 446). Agriculture, he continues in a follow-up piece,

> is treated as a subject so remote from common life, by all those who do not immediately hold the plough, or give fodder to the ox, that I think there is room to question, whether a great part of mankind has yet been informed that life is sustained by the fruits of the earth … . Agriculture, and agriculture alone, can support us without the help of others, in certain plenty, and genuine dignity. Whatever we buy from without, the sellers may refuse; whatever we sell, manufactured by art, the purchasers may reject; but, while our ground is covered with corn and cattle, we can want nothing; and if imagination should grow sick of native plenty, and call for delicacies or embellishments from other countries, there is nothing which corn and cattle will not purchase. (1810b, 451)

Johnson idealizes the imagined self-sufficiency of a Britain growing its own grain and raising its own cattle; he makes no direct reference to cattle plague, but his text was written in the midst of an international outbreak, which, according to Dossie, had been brought to England from the Netherlands in 1744 or 1745, then declined, and "took fresh vigor in 1756" (374). Johnson's remarks, then, suggest an *anxiety* about England's vulnerability to international breakouts, and a renewed interest in the role of the farmer who stands on the front lines in battling what Dossie had called "one of the most heavy calamities that can befall and European country," a "scarcity of horned beasts" (482). Fears about such scarcity are easily channeled into claims about economics, national security and self-sufficiency—what we would call "biosecurity"—and correspondent calls for trade regulation and agricultural reform. Johnson's farmer, with abundant "corn and cattle," protects the nation's body politic as well as its "horned beasts" and agricultural productivity.

In their introduction to a collection on bioinsecurity and vulnerability published before the COVID-19 pandemic, the editors, Nancy Chen and Lesley Sharp, describe biosecurity as an increasingly "mundane aspect of human experience," as a "catchall for the detection, surveillance, containment, and deflection of everything from epidemics and natural disasters to resource scarcities, enabling newly conceived mandates in nation-states" including efforts to "police citizens, migrants, and refugees; to reconfigure urban zones, rural landscapes, and border zones" (2014, xi). Throughout this study, I have focused mostly on food scarcity, climate disruptions, and murrain as key elements of bioinsecurity, but influencing my argument in this chapter and the next is a brilliant 2016 study by Neel Ahuja, who links disease interventions to the government of species. "The greatest error of anthropomorphism," he claims there, "is not that animals or objects are incorrectly attributed human characteristics; it is that those viewed as transparently human are extracted as such from their constitution in a broader domain of biosocial life" (Ahuja 2016, 8). *Those viewed as transparently human* seems an apt description for the assumptions and values that undergird the texts of Johnson, Dossie, Dodd, and Sterne and, more generally, the conceptual, economic, and institutional structures that sustain a fiction of humans as "stable and self-contained," protected from "entanglement with and constitution through other bodies" (8). Although Ahuja traces the logics of biosecurity—and bio*in*security—to US defense circles after World War II, we need to recognize, as I have argued, that complex interventions into the lives of domesticated species occur much earlier and more widely in the history of the West. European countries, visited repeatedly by mysterious diseases that threatened fragile food supplies, developed plague bureaucracies that regulated the movement of humans and animals through borders and roads; instituted certifications of health; and periodically demanded the destruction of large animals who may or may not have been exposed to air, grass, water, or textiles that may or may not have contained noxious poisons, effluvia, fomites, or insects. Dossie even uses the word "*virus*" to describe the active agent in murrain (387). In this context, responses to bioinsecurity become both interventionist and affective. The former, as we have seen, include plague protocols and medical regimes; the latter take various forms. If apocalyptic feelings lead to scourge logic, defensive responses to eco-anxiety abound: minimizing the threat (mocking the King's Speech in 1770), scapegoating others (blame it on the Jacobins), intellectualizing disease rather than acting to contain it (Johnson), deflecting through humor (Sterne), developing reaction formations (the vampire genre, anyone?), lamenting the inevitable (Diggon Davy), or succumbing to neurotic behaviors (virtually everyone in Defoe's works).[14] Given the varied affective responses to a transcorporeal medical disaster that cannot adequately be contained, it is not surprising that the discourse about cattle plague in the eighteenth century seems both diffuse and multilayered. It is the *nature* of anxiety to be indirectly expressed or, just as likely, repressed. If the bovine elegy, along with cattle-centered hymns, offered ways to articulate ecological and biopolitical fears, if it invited readers to entertain a cross-species sensibility and experience shared senses of suffering, the emergent professionalization of literature ensured that these context-specific expressions of grief and loss would fade away—or, be prodded into the margins of an anthropocentric literary culture. The more human humanism becomes, the more difficult it is to recognize the fear and pathos generated by Smit's print, Diggon's lament, or Goldsmith's anger at the plight of poor farmers who must cling to their two or three cows as a fragile bulwark against financial ruin.

References

Ahuja, Neel. 2016. *Bioinsecurities: Disease Interventions, Empire, and the Government of Species*. Durham: Duke University Press.

Annual Register, or a View of the History, Politics, and Literature for the Year 1770. 1785. 4th ed. London: J. Dodsley.

Anon. 1777. *An authentick account of the late unfortunate Doctor William Dodd*. Rochester: Printed by T. Fisher.

Barker, A. D. 1982. The Early Career of William Dodd. *Transactions of the Cambridge Bibliographical Society* 8 (2): 217–235.

Broad, John. 1983. Cattle Plague in Eighteenth-Century England. *Agricultural History Review* 31 (2): 104–115.

Brown, Karen, and Daniel Gilfoyle. 2010. *Healing the Herds: Disease, Livestock Economies, and the Globalization of Veterinary Medicine*. Athens: Ohio University Press.

[14] See Dodds (2021: 222–26).

Brown, Laura. 2017. *Homeless Dogs and Melancholy Apes: Humans and Other Animals in the Modern Literary Imagination*. Ithaca: Cornell University Press.

Brown, Laura. 2023. *The Counterhuman Imaginary: Earthquakes, Lapdogs, and Traveling Coinage in Eighteenth-Century Literature*. Ithaca: Cornell University Press.

Caldwell, Tanya. 2000. *Time to Begin Anew: Dryden's 'Georgics' and 'Aeneis'*. Lewisburg, PA: Bucknell University Press.x.

Caldwell, Tanya. 2008. *Virgil Made English: The Decline of Classical Authority*. London: Palgrave.

Chen, Nancy N., and Lesley A. Sharp, eds. 2014. *Bioinsecurity and Vulnerability*. Albuquerque: University of New Mexico Press.

de Bruyn, Frans. 2005. Eighteenth-Century Editions of Virgil's Georgics: From Classical Poem to Agricultural Treatise. *Lumen* 24:149–163.

Dodd, William. 1767. *Poems by Dr. Dodd*. London: Dryden Leach.

Doddridge, Philip. 1755. *Hymns Founded on Various Texts in the Holy Scriptures*. London: Printed by J. Eddowes and J. Cotton: and sold by J. Waugh and W. Fenner; and J. Buckland.

Dodds, Joseph. 2021. The Psychology of Climate Anxiety. *British Journal of Psychiatry Bulletin* 45 (4): 222–226.

Dossie, Robert. 1771. *Memoirs of Agriculture, and other Oeconomical Arts*, 2 vols. London: J. Nourse.

Dryden, John. 1987. In *The Works of John Dryden, Volume V: Poems 1697*, ed. William Frost. Berkeley: University of California Press.

Faber, J. A. 1962. Cattle-Plague in the Netherlands during the Eighteenth Century. *Mededelingen van de Landbouwhogeschool te Wageningen, Nederland* 62 (11): 1–7.

Fudge, Erica. 2018. *Quick Cattle and Dying Wishes: People and Their Animals in Early Modern England*. Ithaca: Cornell University Press.

Gibbs, F. W. 1951. Robert Dossie (1717–1777) and the Society of Arts. *Annals of Science* 7 (2): 149–172.

Goldsmith, Oliver. 1774. *An History of the earth and animated Nature*, 8 vols. London: J. Nourse.

Griffin, Michael. 2013. *Enlightenment in Ruins: The Geographies of Oliver Goldsmith*. Lewisburg, PA: Bucknell University Press.

Hardwick, Joseph. 2024. Cows, Community, and Religious Responses to the 1865–66 British Rinderpest Outbreak. *Journal of Religious History* 48 (2): 153–171.

Hervey, James. (1796) 1808. *Meditations and Contemplations*, 2 vols. Philadelphia: B. and T. Kite.

Johnson, Samuel. 1810a. Some Thoughts on Agriculture both Ancient and Modern, With an Account of the Honor Due to the English Farmer. In *The Works of Samuel Johnson*, ed. Arthur Murphy, vol. II. London: Luke Hansard and Sons.

Johnson, Samuel. 1810b. Further Thoughts on Agriculture. In *The Works of Samuel Johnson*, ed. Arthur Murphy, vol. II. London: Luke Hansard and Sons.

Koolmees, Peter A. 2010. Epizootic Diseases in the Netherlands, 1713–2002: Veterinary Science, Agricultural Policy, and Public Response. In *Healing the Herds: Disease, Livestock Economies, and the Globalization of Veterinary Medicine*, ed. Karen Brown and Daniel Gilfolye, 19–41. Athens, OH: Ohio University Press.

Kurth, Charlie, and Panu Pihkala. 2022. Eco-anxiety: What It Is and Why It Matters. *Frontiers in Psychology* 13.

Kurzer, Frederick. 2004. Chemistry in the Life of Dr. Samuel Johnson. *Bulletin of the History of Chemistry* 29 (2): 65–88.

Landry, Donna. 2009. *Noble Brutes: How Eastern Horses Transformed English Culture.* Baltimore: Johns Hopkins University Press.

Landry, Donna. 2011. English Brutes, Eastern Enlightenment. *The Eighteenth Century: Theory and Interpretation* 52 (1): 11–30.

Layard, Daniel Peter. 1770. *An essay on the nature, causes, and cure of the contagious distemper among the horned cattle in these kingdoms.* London: J. and F. Rivington.

Lind, James. 1763. *Two papers on fevers and infection: which were read before the Philosophical and Medical Society, in Edinburgh.*

Lobb, Theophilus. 1745. Letter VIII: Relating to Contagious Sicknesses among Cattle. In *Letters Relating to the Plague and other Contagious Distempers*, 382–383. London: James Buckland.

London Gazette 8518. March 11–March 15, 1745.

London Gazette 8623 March 14–March 17, 1746.

Ludovice, Nicolo Paolo. 2021. Covid-19 as a Zoonotic Moment: Placing the Animal at the Forefront of the History of Pandemics. In *Working Papers in Critical Disaster Studies*, Series 1: 2, 1–10. New York: Initiative for Critical Disaster Studies.

MacCallum, David. 2019. *Volcanoes in Eighteenth-Century Europe: An Essay in Environmental Humanities.* Liverpool: Liverpool University Press.

Maehle, A. H. 2013. Four Early Clinical Studies to Assess the Effects of Peruvian Bark. *Journal of the Royal Society of Medicine* 106 (4): 150–155.

Markley, Robert. 1999. Foucault, Modernity, and the Cultural Study of Science. *Configurations: A Journal of Literature, Science, and Technology* 7:153–173.

Mascall, Leonard. 1587. *The First Booke of Cattel.* London: Iohn Wolfe.

Mason, Travis. 2014. 'Having Cleared and Embellished the Earth': Agricultural Science and Poetic Tradition in Oliver Goldsmith's *The Deserted Village. Studies in Canadian Literature/Etudes en Littérature Canadienne* 39 (1): 21–39.

Massey, William. 1865. *A History of England during the Reign of George III.* London: Longman and Greens.

Menely, Tobias. 2006. Animal Signs and Ethical Significance: Expressive Creatures in the British Georgic. *Mosaic: An Interdisciplinary Critical Journal* 39 (4): 111–127.

Menely, Tobias. 2015. *The Animal Claim: Sensibility and the Creaturely Voice.* Chicago: University of Chicago Press.

Mitchell, Robert. 2007. *Sympathy and the State in the Romantic Era: Systems, State Finance, and the Shadows of Futurity.* New York: Routledge.

Mortimer, Cromwell. 1745a. Some Account of the Distemper Raging among the Cow-kind in the Neighborhood of London, together with some Remedies proposed for their Recovery. *Philosophical Transactions of the Royal Society* 43 (477): 532–537.

Mortimer, Charles. 1745b. Further Observations on the Distemper Now Raging among the Cow-Kind, by the Publisher of These Transactions. *Philosophical Transactions* 43 (478): 549–555.

Mortimer, Charles. 1746. A Third Account of the Distemper among the Cows. *Philosophical Transactions* 44 (479): 4–10.

Mullet, Charles F. 1946. The Cattle Distemper in Mid-Eighteenth-Century England. *Agricultural History* 20 (3): 144–165.

Newfield, Timothy P. 2015. Domesticates, Disease and Climate in Early Post-Classical Europe: The Cattle Plague of c.940 and Its Environmental Context. *Postclassical Archaeologies* 5:95–126.

Parisot, Eric. 2015. The Work of Feeling in James Hervey's Mediations among the Tombs (1746). *Parergon* 31 (2): 121–135.

Patel, Raj, and Jason Moore. 2018. *The History of the World in Seven Cheap Things: Capitalism, Nature, and the Future of the Planet.* Berkeley: University of California Press.

Porter, Natalie M. 2019. *Viral Economies: Bird Flu Experiments in Vietnam.* Chicago: University of Chicago Press.

Ritvo, Harriet. 1989. *The Animal Estate: The English and Other Creatures in Victorian England.* Cambridge, MA: Harvard University Press.

Spilsbury, Francis. 1785a. *The Power of Gold Displayed: In the Humane Proposal of the Right Hon. William Pitt, Chancellor of the Exchequer, to Bring Forward an Act to put His Majesty into the Disagreeable Situation of Signing a Decree, that no Sick or Lame person, or Diseased Cattle … shall have a Medicine of Repute without Paying Tribute.* London: Sold at the Dispensary, Soho Square.

Spilsbury, Francis. 1785b. *The New Medicine Act Considered, as Now Substituted in the House of Commons, July 8, 1785. Published with The Power of Gold Displayed.* London: Sold at the Dispensary, Soho Square.

Spinage, C. A. 2003. *Cattle Plague: A History.* Amsterdam: Kluwer Academic/ Plenum Publishers.

Stebbings, Chantal. 2014. Tax and Quacks: The Policy of the Eighteenth-Century Medicine Stamp Duty. In *Studies in the History of Tax Law*, ed. J. Tiley, vol. 6. Oxford: Hart Publishing.

Sterne, Laurence. 1788. *Original Letters of the Late Reverend Mr. Laurence Sterne*. Comp. William Combe. Dublin: Printed for H. Chamberlaine, et al.

Thomas, Keith. 1983. *Man and the Natural World: Changing Attitudes in England 1500–1800*. London: Allen Lane.

Thomas, Peter D. G. 1996. *John Wilkes, A Friend to Liberty*. Oxford: Oxford University Press.

Valenze, Deborah. 2006. *The Social Life of Money in the English Past*. Cambridge: Cambridge University Press.

Van Renen, Denys. 2023. 'Eternal Sunshine': Intertexuality as Environmental History in Oliver Goldsmith's *The Deserted Village*. *Studies in Eighteenth-Century Culture* 52:467–475.

White, Sam. 2010. Rethinking Disease in Ottoman. *International Journal of Middle East Studies* 42 (4): 549–567.

White, Sam. 2011. *The Climate of Rebellion in the Early Modern Ottoman Empire*. Cambridge: Cambridge University Press.

Wilkinson, Lise. 1992. *Animals and Disease: An Introduction to the History of Comparative Medicine*. Cambridge: Cambridge University Press.

Wolloch, Nathaniel. 2006. *Subjugated Animals: Animals and Anthropocentrism in Early Modern European Culture*. Amherst, NY: Prometheus Books.

Wood, Gillen. 2014. *Tambora: The Eruption that Changed the World*. Princeton: Princeton University Press.

CHAPTER 6

Steppe Disease and Cholera During Britain's Last Great Outbreak, 1865–1866

Abstract In 1865 and 1866, after a series of outbreaks on the continent, cattle plague returned to England. In contrast to eighteenth-century writers, as Lyon Playfair's 1866 *The Cattle Plague in its Relation to Past Epidemics and to the Present Attack* attests, many nineteenth-century physicians and politicians brought to cattle plague knowledge about infection and sanitary practices gained through a century of fighting cholera outbreaks in human populations. Although reprising many of the discourses featured in previous chapters (insects as disease vectors, the bovine elegy, and pastoral politics), this chapter focuses on the constitutive functions of an analogy between cholera and rinderpest. On the one hand, drawing on lessons from cholera, the sanitary movement advocated for better conditions (clean water, mucked stalls, roomier train cars) for cattle raised or transported to market; on the other hand, cattle became more deeply embedded in the imperial logics of import theory and steppe disease—the belief that "foreign" cattle or "alien" husbandry practices, rather than the local cattle market or a divinely-sanctioned meat-based diet, were responsible for epizootics and panzootics. I end this chapter by discussing what is perhaps the only British novel on rinderpest, Sophie Amelia Prosser's 1872 *The Days of the Cattle Plague*.

L. Cole, *The Fifth Plague*, Palgrave Studies in Animals and Literature, https://doi.org/10.1007/978-3-031-92793-5_6

Medicine has never shown great powers of cure in cases of great plagues.
Lyon Playfair, *The Cattle Plague in its Relation to Past Epidemics and to the Present Attack* (1866)

By 1842, when memories of England's eighteenth-century cattle plagues had begun to recede, the British government abolished all prohibitions against the importation of cattle, abandoning disease control in the name of free trade (Fisher 1980, 278–294). This *laissez faire* attitude almost immediately resulted in outbreaks of foot and mouth disease, pleuropneumonia, and other illnesses, although rinderpest—the scourge of the eighteenth century—did not return to Great Britain until June of 1865 (Spinage 2003, 272). Despite repeated cautions by John Gamgee, the noted Scots veterinarian, who had been warning various public bodies about the dangers of importing cattle since 1863, Britain found itself, again, in the throes of a devastating outbreak (Hall 1962, 45–58). The number of cases of infected cattle doubled every four weeks for months. The Privy Council, faced with no operative means to arrest the plague, and without naming it "rinderpest," issued an anemic Order of Council in July, leveling a small fine against cattle owners in the Metropolitan Market who failed to report diseased cattle. This action was followed by a second order on August 11 that employed the more ominous term "Cattle Plague," and then by a host of bills proposed, withdrawn, amended, and consolidated throughout 1865. Yet by the end of that year 73,549 animals, according to Sherwin Hall, had been infected, of which 41,495 died, and 13,931 had been slaughtered (Hall, 45). Finally, in February of 1866, the *Cattle Diseases Prevention Act 1866* made it through both houses of Parliament. Diseased animals were to be slaughtered and buried, cattle owners would be compensated, and local inspectors would be appointed to ensure compliance. In the wake of its passage, two scientific or epidemiological questions and several policy issues dominated discussions of, and controversies about, the *Cattle Diseases Prevention Act*: whether cattle plague was imported or of "spontaneous generation"—a debate often framed as "contagionism" versus "anti-contagionism"—and whether diseased cows should be culled or cured.

Criticisms of both the government and the medical profession during this crisis were plentiful, loud, and contradictory. To offer two examples: in February of 1866, *Punch, or the London Charivari* ridiculed government action—or inaction—in a full-page cartoon featuring a suffering bovine, "The Patient," surrounded by "cow-doctors" who, indifferent to the dying animal, argue among themselves. The cow laments, "Oh, if

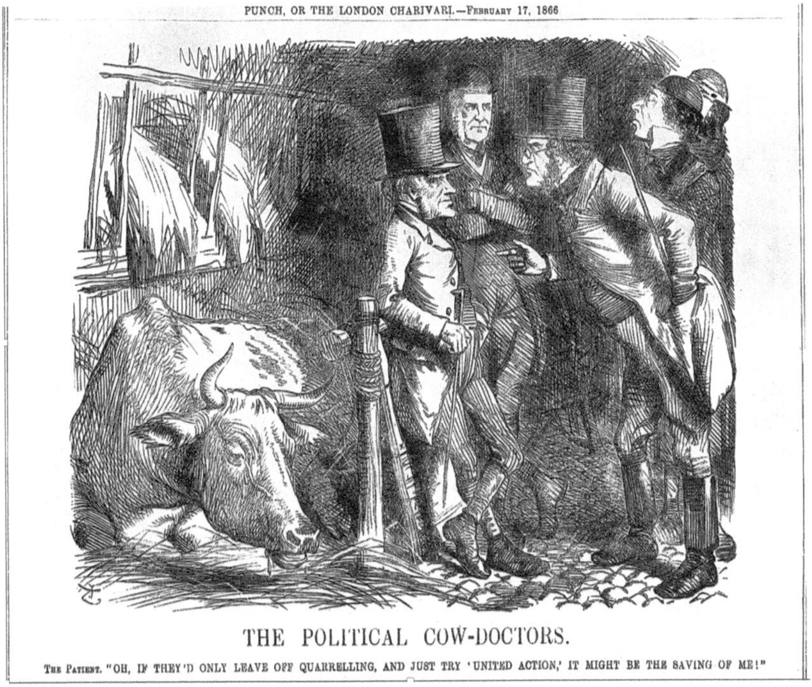

Fig. 6.1 "The Political Cow-Doctors." *Punch; or the London Charivari* (February 17, 1866)

they'd only leave off quarrelling, and just try 'united action,' it might be the saving of me!" (1866a, 69). By displacing blame onto these "quarrelling" veterinarians, the cartoon gestures to supporting a strong national plan—the same plan that many of Punch's readers opposed on economic grounds (Fig. 6.1).

The contradictory position of *Punch* becomes more explicit in the March 3 issue, which contains a poem called "Bos Locutus" ("The Ox Speaks"). Now the ox voices frustration with government interference. It begins

> Pity the sorrows of a poor old Cow
> With Rinderpest a-knocking at the door,
> And what's far worse, these Acts that won't allow
> A chance for life, e'en if the plague's got o'er. (1866b, 87)

Subsequent stanzas lament the loss of English "self-government" under the new Council Orders, which are to "Slay, isolate, stamp out!"—in other words, to employ the traditional methods of culling and quarantine. The ox complains about regulations on movement—"Forbade to change a field, or cross a road, / Fined if we move, and if we linger, slain"—and then about laws restricting imports and exports:

> If foreigners, doomed where we land, to die;
> If natives, when we're sick, debarr'd from cure;
> No medi'cine but the pole-axe let to try –
> A remedy at once too sharp and sure! (1866b, 87)

The target of the poem, unlike the cartoon, is not disputatious veterinarians but Parliament, criticized for failing to act quickly. "Months since, perhaps," it continues, "one effort sharp and strong,/ Had stamped the plague out," but Parliament dawdled, and now it is too late:

> You had halted between 'kill or cure' so long,
> The case has grown past cure, howe'er you kill.
> And when the pest, sown broadcast, wide had spread,
> To panic from paralysis you swing;
> And to the Cattle plague the steppes have bred.
> Add all the cattle-plagues your Act must bring. (87)

Because the government, alternating between "panic and paralysis," cannot decide between "kill or cure," it becomes responsible in this poem for the consequences of infection. The pandemic is as deadly in its own way as the cattle plague supposedly bred on the Russian "steppes."

Punch's satires of the cattle plague controversies provide a glimpse of the fevered political atmosphere during the 1866 outbreak. While historians have done valuable work in exploring the positions in the veterinary debate—contagionism versus anti-contagionism, cull versus cure—I want to focus in this chapter on one issue missing from most histories of cattle plague in the 1860s: a constitutive analogy between "steppe disease" and cholera.[1] I realize that, from the perspective of veterinary history, both typhus and smallpox are more obvious comparisons. As I noted in the last chapter, Peter Layard's *An Essay on the Nature, Causes, and Cure of the*

[1] On cholera and rinderpest, see Spinage (2003, 328–29), and on constitute analogy in science, see Stepan (1986, 261–277).

Contagious Distemper among the Horned Cattle in These Kingdoms (1757) makes a sustained case for analogies between smallpox and rinderpest, a similarity, as we shall see, that helps ground Lyon Playfair's argument for rinderpest vaccination.[2] Yet cholera also offered a powerful pathological model for European physicians struggling to treat a devastating cattle disease: like rinderpest, cholera was characterized by fatal bouts of diarrhea, and—because vaccinations against rinderpest had not proved widely successful—cholera also provided a different conceptual model from smallpox: widespread policies to contain outbreaks. This analogy was recognized at the time by some physicians and veterinarians. Measures to combat cholera, writes the French physician Honoré Bourguignon, give "us a scale by which we may estimate the efforts which will be made to arrest the generation and the contagion of the cattle typhus" (Bourguignon 1869, 214). By "scale" he invokes the international cooperation undertaken to curtail pilgrimages to cholera-stricken Mecca; in 1865, Europe and the Ottoman Empire coordinated efforts to institute a vast quarantine and sanitary system in the lands bordering the Red Sea to curtail the spread of the disease (Mishra 2011a, 53–80).

The analogy between cholera and rinderpest was motivated by the same anxiety about *movement* and transmission of disease that led writers in the sixteenth century to speculate on the role of locusts in spreading contagion and, as late as the early eighteenth century, to perceive insects as a visual analogue for the spread of cattle plague. In the nineteenth century, cholera and rinderpest were tethered by virtue of the widespread belief that plagues must be "imported" from an "uncivilized" elsewhere—India in the case of cholera, the steppes of central and western Asia in the case of rinderpest. The international spread of these diseases, according to many advocates for contagionism, demanded that European nations needed to coordinate efforts to battle these "alien" threats.[3] Between 1745, the year of England's previous major outbreak of rinderpest, and 1865, Great Britain suffered three major cholera epidemics (in the 1830s,

[2]The secondary literature on cowpox, smallpox, and vaccination is extensive. A succinct introduction can be found in Snowden (2019, 83–110). On smallpox and literature, see Shuttleton (2007, 152, 182–184, 200–202). On smallpox and cattle disease, see Spinage (416–422).

[3]A significant body of work exists on colonialism and public health in the nineteenth century. In addition to Mishra (2011a), see Mishra (2011b); Mishra (2011c); Otis (1999); Bashford (2003); Kolb (2021); Servitje (2021); and, on animals and colonial power, Hevia (2018).

1840s, and 1860s) and France, Germany, and the United States were affected as well (Gilbert 2009, Delaporte 1986, Evans 1987, Rosenberg 1962). Britons also were well aware of the gruesome toll of the disease in South Asia. Cholera and famine killed upward of 20,000,000 in India, disproportionately among the poor and undernourished (Arnold 1986, 118–151). Like cholera, cattle plague by the mid-nineteenth century was firmly identified with a specific geographic and geopolitical origin, reflected in names familiar to readers of medical journals as well as the popular press: "Siberian pest," or "steppe disease." To imagine cholera as a foreign disease "imported" into Europe minimizes—at least ideologically—the role that the British empire played in its spread, even as millions in South Asia were immiserated by the economic vice-grip of land policies and taxation, and cholera outbreaks were exacerbated by colonial railway systems and large-scale troop movements in India (Davis 2000). Similarly, transnational movements of goods, peoples, animals, and animal products, especially from breeding and grazing pastures of the steppes, accelerated the incidence of livestock diseases in England and fueled the belief that livestock cattle disease necessarily came from the East. Lyon Playfair, then Professor of Chemistry at the University of Edinburgh and vice-president of the Royal Society of Edinburgh, readily admits that the "completion of the two great lines of railway which, traversing Southern and Central Germany, connect Rotterdam and Hamburg with Pesth and Lemberg, have opened up to us the supplies of Hungary and Galacia, and have vastly increased the danger of a constant importation of this plague" (1866, 20). The notion of an alien origin, then, becomes a way of organizing (often racist) attitudes toward livestock disease and justifying protectionist policies, even as it marginalizes Europe's role in this imperial and epidemiological feedback loop.

Although we now know that cholera is caused by bacteria and rinderpest by a morbillivirus, the nineteenth-century comparisons between them fall into two overlapping groups: the first based on similar progressions of disease or morbid anatomy, the second grounded in policy arguments about how to mitigate their devastating effects. In the first part of this chapter, I lay out some of the nineteenth-century medical arguments for linking cholera, or sometimes typhus, to rinderpest, relying mostly on texts forged in the early months of the outbreak. In line with the values and assumptions of the sanitary movement, these texts recommend a wide array of preventative and curative practices—including slaughter and ingested pesticides, but also hot-air baths, healthy diets, and, in the case of

William Budd, disinfected manure. The next section focuses on Honoré Bourguignon's 1869 treatise *On the Cattle Plague; or Contagious Typhus in Horned Cattle*, a lengthy historically—and experimentally—informed argument for combining stamp-out policies with husbandry practices that could mitigate the consequences of what he calls an "epizootic genius." In France, rinderpest was known as the typhus *contagieux des bêtes á cornes* (Playfair, 21). The steppe cattle are not, Bourguignon argues, intrinsically defective (as other writers suggest), but susceptible to "specific morbific causes," including extreme variations in seasons, that would affect cattle anywhere, including France, given similar conditions and treatment. In his text, the "steppes" offer an example of the kind of neglectful husbandry that European farmers are enjoined to reject both medically and morally. Bourguignon's version of pastoral politics, updated for an increasingly industrialized cattle industry, is reflected in the *Cattle Diseases Prevention Act 1866*, which I explore in the next section. Playfair, a member of the Cattle Act Commission and one of the authors of the Act, was a well-known advocate for the sanitary movement. In his *The Cattle Plague in its Relation to Past Epidemics and to the Present Attack* (1866), Playfair claims that mitigation measures in the 1860s are superior to those adopted during the 1745 plague, yet he remains pessimistic about their ability to stop what he perceives as a plague imported from the steppes. The contagionist debates in the 1860s produced a variety of texts that went beyond veterinary disputes, and to conclude this chapter I discuss two of most revealing: H. Strickland Constable's satirical response to the 1866 Cattle Act, a sinkhole of plague disinformation, and a popular religious novel, *The Days of the Cattle Plague* (1872). The latter, by Sophie Amelia Prosser, refurbishes providentialist readings of livestock disease, even as it endorses the measures taken by Queen Victoria's government.

"Bovine Stink" and the Sanitary Movement

Throughout the nineteenth century, the world was pummeled by a series of disease outbreaks in both humans and animals. Finally and unequivocally, a rapidly professionalizing medical field demonstrated a keen interest in exploring relations between them (Bynum 1994; Weisz 2003: 536–575; Burney 2007, 46–57). In 1862, the British Medical Association passed a resolution "binding the Association," writes William Budd, "to take up at once the study of epidemic and epizootic diseases" (Budd 1865a, 169n). Long before that resolution, however, comparative pathology was increasingly common in medical writing, and the desire to establish links between epidemics and epizootics, especially "steppe disease" or "the Siberian pest," became a regular feature in discussions of contagious disease. According to Thomas Southwood Smith, the physician and sanitary reformer, London's cholera outbreak in 1831 coincided with "diseases of the lower animals – horses, cows, sheep, and all domestic creatures," possibly the result of a shared cause in the "peculiar epidemic constitution of the air" (Smith 1866, 2).[4] In the 1850s, when the founder of modern epidemiology, John Snow, first traced a London cholera outbreak to the Broad Street pump, *The Lancet, The British Medical Journal*, and other medical venues in Britain and Ireland published a series of articles by William Lauder Lindsay and fellow physicians on the relationships between "steppe disease" and cholera.[5] Like cholera, according to Lindsay, rinderpest is "essentially a fever": both diseases involve "collapse," followed by "excitement of the system," or diarrhea; after nine days, both diseases exhibit "pustules" and, in some cases, respiratory difficulties; and both are "incurable, intensely contagious, and very fatal, the deaths amounting to from fifty to ninety per cent" (1857, 496–97). Although admitting that there is not yet proof that the diseases are identical, Lindsay points out that the resemblance is so striking that "various authors" describe "*choleraic* diarrhoeah" (497) as the final stage of rinderpest, preceding death. Recounting his own experiments on cholera in dogs, he advocates for more experimentation on "diseases transmissible between man and animals" as well as those "occurring coincidently with epidemics in man" (499), notably cholera and steppe disease.

William Budd's address to the annual meeting of the British Medical Association in August 1865 was entitled "The Siberian Cattle Plague; or, the Typhoid Fever of the Ox." Typhus was "so widely supported" as the cause of the disease at the beginning of the 1865 outbreak that "it was almost a matter of common belief" (Spinage, 9). Although both smallpox and typhoid fever were also analogical candidates, cholera was a contagious disease that could be mitigated by sanitary measures. Budd's commitment to sanitary reform structures his address and offers a means to analyze the logic of those advocates who believed Britain could control cattle plague through improved hygienic measures. Maintaining that

[4] On Smith's career, see Cook (2002: 194–205).

[5] *The Dublin Quarterly Journal of Medical Science* 42 (1866), 137. In this review, published under the title "Work on Cholera," the author reviews eight texts on the disease.

cattle plague spreads largely through aerosolized fecal matter and groundwater contamination, Budd begins his address by emphasizing that humans and animals are "preyed upon by a great and fatal brood of specific diseases"; because we are "so truly members of one family," some diseases "pass entire" across species. Among such diseases he names human smallpox and sheep smallpox, Asiatic cholera, plague, scarlet fever, yellow fever, lung disease in cattle, and typhoid and typhus fevers as the "leading types of this great Army of Death." Rinderpest, he asserts, "bear[s] the closest family resemblance to human typhoid" (169), and, like typhoid fever and "Asiatic cholera," is spread through "specific germs" in drinking water. Consequently, improved drainage and the careful disposal of waste products, in his view, are among the best defenses against a wide range of human and animal diseases (178).

Despite the scientific evidence Budd marshals to support his argument, he nonetheless falls back on scapegoating alien peoples, climates, and cultures for the ills of the West. He describes the Siberian steppes as the source of rinderpest and "still its great stronghold." His language is redolent with the rhetoric, assumptions, and values of nineteenth-century sanitary science. "Somewhere or another in that wide area," he claims,

> which looks so blank on our maps, now in sporadic, now in epizootic form, [the disease] is always present. In these wild wastes, this fell disorder works its will on the hapless and unconscious cattle, unchecked by veterinary police or sanitary reformer. There is no Farr there to point, in words of real wisdom, the moral of pestilence; no Chadwick to preach a crusade against bovine stinks; no Florence Nightingale to teach physicians that contagion is an antiquated myth; no Murchison to commit himself to the hopeless task of showing that, although essentially contagious, this typhoid fever of the ox is caused, for the most part, by putrid faeces, or, in one word, a pythogenic fever. (169)

Budd creates a lineage for his treatise that includes the work of leading researchers on cholera and voices of moral as well as medical authority. William Farr was the first person to compare local mortality rates and adjust for differences among sub-groups and towns, a refinement that allowed him to track down the source of cholera to contaminated water supplies. Edwin Chadwick's *Report on the Sanitary Condition of the Population of Great Britain* (1842) led to legislation that promoted cleaner water and more efficient waste removal. Florence Nightingale advocated clean air and fresh water in hospitals during the Crimean War, and Charles Murchison coined the term "filth diseases" to describe infections in the gastrointestinal and respiratory tracts, including bubonic plague, dysentery, and typhoid, as well as scabies and ringworm. For Murchison, "filth diseases" stem from the horrid living conditions of the poor and must be combatted by sanitary reform.

Armed with the values and assumptions of the sanitation movement, Budd describes the steppes as a seething pit of contagion. "Under the rapid evaporation which often prevails in the open Steppe," he argues, "intestinal discharges" of infected cattle must "occur on a very large scale"; desiccated, infected feces become airborne as "impalpable dust . . . in the great company of other infected germs" (174). He invokes a Russian Government report that notes the "dung of some diseased oxen, which had lain for months under the snow and ice of a Russian winter" (170) remained infectious. Trade and war, "those two inexorable tyrants," drive the "fatal and characteristic power of migration": "vast droves" of cattle leave the steppes "for the markets of the west," carrying with them "the germs of the scourge" that provoke "great outbreaks," with victims numbering in the "tens of thousands" (169). The persistent diarrhea that characterizes cattle disease "taint[s] the soil on which the patient stands," and then "the ship, the wharf, the cattle truck, the public road, and the market" (174). Eventually, "like those of cholera and human typhoid" these discharges taint groundwater, leading to what appear to unscientifically inclined observers as local, environmental outbreaks traceable to local conditions. Budd advocates three strategies of prevention: slaughtering infected cattle; deploying *cordon sanitaires* in eastern and central Europe to prevent "reimportation of the pest"; and, significantly, eliminating "all poison cast off by [infected cattle]" (178). His recommendations, in this respect, go beyond providing access to clean drinking water and effective drainage: "The most direct and effectual way" to halt the spread of disease, he contends, "is to destroy those germs immediately on their issue from body," before infected feces reach the drains, a practice that had been deployed since 1859 to prevent both typhoid fever and "Asiatic cholera" (178). For Budd, the disaster of "Asiatic cholera" offers a compelling case for implementing strict national quarantine policies and better hygienic practices.

The steppes, correspondingly, offer a kind of epidemiological cautionary tale about infection and airborne transmission of dried fecal matter. Budd's characterization of the steppes as a "blank space on a map" is, of course, an imperial metaphor that obscures two centuries of Western Europeans using Central Asian and Eastern European grasslands as breeding ground and pasture for livestock imported, fattened, and butchered closer to home. As I argued in Chap. 4, "Tartars" and the steppes had been the subject of western fear and fascination throughout the eighteenth century. In the nineteenth, Central Asia and Siberia became increasingly integrated into western-dominated international trade and even began to attract western tourists. Lucy Sherrard Atkinson, an English governess in Moscow, traveled with her husband, Thomas Witlam Atkinson, some 40,000 miles across the steppes between 1848 and 1853; her 1863 account of this journey, *Recollections of Tartar Steppes and Their Inhabitants* (Fig. 6.2), recounts both vast herding practices and colonial mining operations. The so-called blankness of the steppes, then, is really an invitation to demonize an epidemiological other, a space of excremental "filth" and unchecked plague, where infection is allowed to "steal, unheeded, far and wide, through the land" (Budd 1865a 170).

Also in 1865, other pieces on cholera and cattle plague began to appear side-by-side in the *British Medical Journal*, more or less taking for granted Budd's argument that because rinderpest and cholera are alike, their spread can be mitigated by sanitary science. Which particular strategy, or

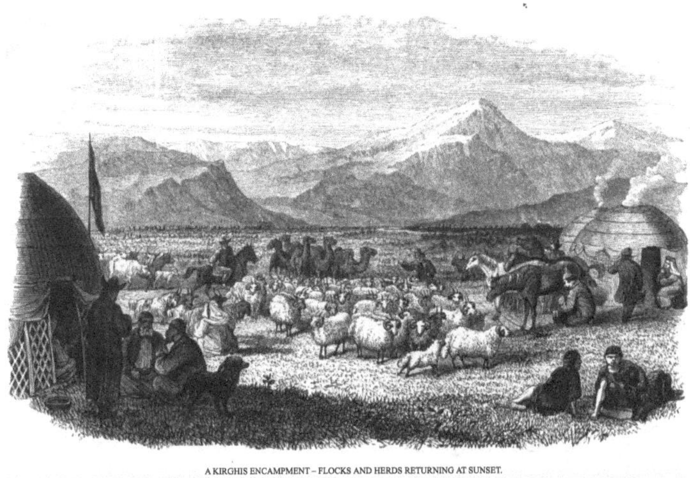

A KIRGHIS ENCAMPMENT – FLOCKS AND HERDS RETURNING AT SUNSET.

Fig. 6.2 Frontispiece to Lucy Atkinson's *Recollections of Tartar Steppes and Their Inhabitants* (London: John Murray, 1863). Public domain

strategies, of sanitary science should be deployed, however, remained a subject of intense debate. On September 16, James Gardner, a colonial medical officer, warned that the "spreading of cholera on the continent, the presence of zymotic diseases, the disease amongst cattle, all show that it is not at all unlikely we may yet have a visit from cholera in an epidemic form" (1865, 282). By "zymotic diseases," Gardner means acute infectious diseases characterized by fevers, a group that includes typhus, smallpox, and cholera. The term carries with it traces of miasma theory; in the words of the physician Daniel Holt, this "class" of diseases implies that a "morbid principle or miasm" has entered the nervous system, blood, and tissues, eventually affecting "the system generally" (Holt 1856, 370). By linking cholera, cattle disease, and fevers, Gardner treats them as part of a general pestilential condition that requires "adopt[ing] strict hygienic measures," including cleanliness, healthy diets, and improved drainage systems, especially in low-lying areas. "If everyone were to adopt such measures," Gardner maintains, there would be "no such thing as cholera or any other infectious disease known"; people who ignore such strictures "succumb to the disease [and] then propagate it to their neighbors" (282–283). The difference between a clean and healthy environment in England and alien "filth diseases," spreading unchecked on the steppes, is projected back onto medical debates: the advocates and practitioners of sanitary science set against their willfully ignorant or almost sociopathic "neighbors," wallowing in filth.

In the same year, James Tucker, a medical officer in Ireland, published his *Essay on the Nature and Treatment of Cholera and Fever, with Medical Remarks on the Treatment of Cattle Plague*, which contained an appendix on "Public Health." He makes explicit what Gardner implies: that "cholera, fevers, and the typhoid fever of cattle – the Siberian plague – [...] are members of one family of zymotic or fermentable disorders," traceable to "one common fosterer": "We inhale these pestilential germs in foul air, and drink them in foul water" (Tucker 1865, 5). Citing microscopist Dr. Lionel Beale, Tucker calls these entities "particles of living germinal matter" that, once introduced into the body, may either "grow, multiply, give rise to a particular form of disease," or, if introduced into a "healthy organism" (5) that can fight off the infection, may die. He calls on physicians to "extinguish these maladies in the light of sanitary science" (6), largely by exposing cattle to saline waters and hot-air baths.[6] Pitting himself against continental veterinarians and their British counterpart, John Gamgee, who maintained that culling was the only real option for infected cattle, Tucker represents himself as the voice of scientific modernity: "We are on the threshold of great sanitary science. It is not in this age that surgeons of any class should consign their patients to slaughter" (5). His language illustrates how debates about cattle disease resonate with efforts to protect human health and with the discourses of progress, evidence-based science, and national welfare.

Budd's and Tucker's pamphlets were written by physicians, but a third full-length argument, *The Human Blight and Cattle Blight, Or an Explanation of the Cholera and Cattle Plague*, also appeared in August 1866, at the height of the rinderpest outbreak. Publishing anonymously, its author begins by admitting that he is not a "professor of physic"; although, he concedes, *ne sutor ultra crepidam* ("shoemaker, not beyond thy shoe") is generally an "excellent maxim," he argues that because cattle disease is at present "no man's land," he intends to approach the subject with "the common rules of observation and meaning" (1866, a2v) and to recommend common-sense solutions. Like Gardener and Tucker—but unlike Budd—the author describes cholera and rinderpest as seemingly curable. He attributes Tucker's "pestilential germs" and Gardener's "zymotic diseases" to "animalculae"—insects or eggs of insects that "come from the regions of the East," then settle on "the mucus of the intestines, and ultimately the intestines" (5) of cattle and men. In the same way that apple and pear trees have their own pests, he insists, there is one blight for the "bovine" and one for the "human tribe" (7). In both cases, though, the eggs either "germinate and breed inside the animal" or spread "from the excrement of the animals; and thus each animal becomes a center of fresh infection" (7). Through expelled fecal matter, the disease "gathers strength from each victim" (6). If cholera is less fatal to humans than rinderpest is to cattle, that is largely, he suggests, because men eat cooked food, and the heat destroys many of these "animalculae."

Much like Richard Bradley's *The Plague at Marseilles Consider'd*, discussed in Chap. 4, *The Human Blight and the Cattle Blight* walks a fine line between the whimsical and the scientific—at least from the perspective of germ theory. On the one hand, the text admits that we know little

[6] Tucker also wrote a treatise (1860) on how roman "thermo-electrical baths" are "temples of health" for both humans and cattle.

about the "nature of the insects whose attack causes the diseases," and correctly identifies water as a common medium of infection for both cholera and rinderpest:

> The cattle disease has especially been observed to follow the course of streams; the cattle on the stream apparently imbibe the eggs of the blight. When no other means of contagion is discoverable, and in times of the cholera, the outbreak in certain districts is clearly traceable to particular wells. (23–24)

Without naming John Snow, *The Human Blight and the Cattle Blight* mentions how some years ago the "Golden Square" in London was devastated by cholera traced to a particular well. On the other hand, the "cures" promoted by the anonymous author are, at best, dubious: "The true mode of treating the disease in man," the author writes, "and the only mode of treating it in animals, is to introduce into the stomach of the victim a drug which shall poison and kill the insect blight while yet in the stomach, and thus enable the digestive powers of the man or animal to deal with the dead insect blight as it would any other kind of food" (30). Having described the infectious agent as a kind of insect, the author offers insecticides as a cure, notably *assafoetida,* often called "devil's dung" in English, a traditional cure for cholera in India and one highly toxic to mosquito larvae.[7] But, the author continues, any insect poison will do, either as a cure or a preventative. The "proper remedy" for the treatment of cholera is "the strongest insect poison which is compatible with the preservation of human life," and the "preventative" is "whatever keeps the stomach in such a condition as to destroy the eggs of the insects as soon as they are swallowed" (14). What is good for man is good for cattle too: "Observe what is ordinarily deadly to insect life, and adapt it to the internal use of animals" (14). Rhetorically, if not scientifically, readers have entered the realm of speculative analogy: a precursor to hydroxychloroquine and ivermectin as supposed remedies for COVID-19.

In October 1866, the *British Medical Journal* included a short notice of *The Human Blight and Cattle Blight*, referring to the author's description of cattle plague as "no man's land": "As the professional knowledge fails, the anonymous writer concludes that non-professional knowledge may be able to explain the case. The reasoning is curious, and enables one

[7] See Muturi et al. (2019: 337).

to judge, without reading, the character of his argument, and the value of it" (1866, 301: 388). This quick dismissal, justified from an experimental perspective, nonetheless was symptomatic of a growing divide between "official" medical knowledge, represented by the *Lancet* and the *British Medical Journal*, and a host of popular publications that sought to promote "general observation" over specialized scientific knowledge and medical training. Questions about the transmission of zoonotic disease—even when taken almost for granted by Budd and others—irrevocably are caught up in debates about professionalization, scientific authority, and experimental evidence.

"Epizootic Genius"

Michael Worboys has claimed that the failure of veterinarians to find a cure during the 1865 cattle plague lent credence to the default position that animal diseases were imported (1991: 308–327). But the importation thesis and accompanying colonial plague bureaucracies likely were fueled, at least in part, by the experiences of cholera epidemics. In 1865 Honoré Bourguignon's English version of *On the Cattle Plague* issued a call for action based on the presence of a double threat: "To-day," he writes, "we are called upon to resist the baleful effects of cattle typhus, but, [even now] cholera hovers about us. If we do nothing, if we talk and debate instead of acting, these scourges will come upon us on a sudden, and find us quite as helpless as ever to resist their sway" (71). By "acting" Bourguignon means developing and enforcing international (rather than simply national) rules for stopping the movements of people and animals during epizootic outbreaks. "It is well known," he claims, "that the cholera of the present day"

> had its origins on the banks of the Red Sea, amidst the infectious miasmata developed near Mecca, where thousands of pilgrims who had died of fatigue and privation, and hundreds of thousands of sheep butchered and religiously offered up in sacrifice, have, beneath a torrid heat, generated the choleraic miasma, which formerly was supposed to be produced exclusively on the banks of the Ganges. (213)

Bourguignon deploys a by-now familiar litany of causal relations for the cholera outbreak: a climate of "torrid heat," "infectious miasmata," rotting corpses of humans and animals breeding water-borne and airborne disease. In Bourguignon's mind, cholera and rinderpest are linked, and measures to combat cholera offer a means to "estimate the efforts which will be made to arrest the generation and the contagion of the cattle typhus" (214), namely, European cooperation to curtail pilgrimages to Mecca (Mishra 2011b). Bourguignon (who advocates completely prohibiting the Hajj) asks, "why not take the same measures against typhus which are judged necessary against cholera?" (214n).

In the same way cholera can be traced to Mecca, cattle disease originates on the steppes, and Bourguignon rejects both simple contagionist arguments (steppe cattle constitute a tainted "race," and therefore should be kept from England's shores) and anti-contagionist counters (cattle disease can arise spontaneously anywhere, such as London's dairies, where filthy conditions may trigger outbreaks). Instead, he argues that contagious diseases affecting both humans and animals must be considered in the context of "epizootic genius": "a particular state of the atmospheric elements, or the air, . . . whose morbific properties vary in their degree of intensity" (112). In the tropics, he maintains, "an infinity of worms, maggots, animalculae, insects, mollusca, fish, reptiles, birds . . . die and decay," producing a "slime" which then dries and disintegrates to create a "pestiferous vapor" (97). Equally unhealthy conditions can be found "in many parts of the globe" and are especially prevalent in "large tracts of country which are still uninhabited, whose uncultivated soil supplies with food great numbers of sheep and cattle" (14–15), especially Russia, Hungary, Australia, and North and South America. Seasonal weather brings "rich and luxuriant verdure," enabling animals to withstand long, arduous journeys "and to supply the rich countries of the West with their flesh, fleece, and hides" (16). But because there is little "foresight" or good husbandry in these areas, cattle suffer when the seasons change to floods or scorching sun:

> hard is their fate under the pressing need of hunger. Peaceful creatures, they browse in vain on deleterious plants on a sterile soil; their external and internal teguments now afford a favourable seat for the propagations of parasites—for the *parasitogenia*; and soon after a general *adynamia*, or relaxation of the fibres, delivers them up without resistance to the morbific elements of the infectious diseases to which they are exposed, where the languishing, the sick, and the rotting are herded together, and they are carried off by hecatombs by this wasteful and devouring typhus. (17–18)

Plagues in the Bible and those alluded to by Homer, Plutarch, Virgil, and Ovid, he claims, resemble "the epidemics or plagues which are witnessed in our own day" (20). Nineteenth-century countries with harsh environmental conditions, in brief, replicate the outmoded practices and beliefs of ancient cultures in recognizing, or failing to recognize, factors that lead to endemic cattle disease.

For Bourguignon, then, the 1865 outbreak in England can also be attributed to "epizootic genius" exacerbated by poor husbandry practices. Anywhere there is "some violent change of season, such as extreme droughts, or superabundant rains" (112) as in 1864 and 1865, when "excessive drought [persisted] in various parts of Europe," (113) the decline in the quality and quantity of pasture can kickstart a cycle of livestock scrounging for "deleterious plants" (114). England suffered more than any other country; abundance turned to scarcity, and large herds of cattle wandered from field to field seeking "for something to browse on a parched and arid soil" (114). Under such circumstances, the vital resistance of English livestock deteriorated, and they became, like steppe cattle, more susceptible to disease. In this manner, he argues, "we may account for and reconcile the two contending theories, one of which refers the cause of this typhus to foreign importation, whilst the other insists that it originated in the filthy and half-ventilated cowsheds of the metropolis" (117). In brief, he offers what he believes is an explanation that transcends contemporary debates about anti-contagionism and contagionism, between advocates for killing and quarantining sick animals and the proponents of sanitary science.

To recognize and value the impact of "epizootic genius" on human and animal plagues requires a new kind of medicine and a new pastoral politics. Bourguignon insists on the importance of comparative medicine on moral as well as scientific grounds. In ways that evoke both Exodus and Lucretius, he glosses over differences between human and animal plagues to focus on their resemblances, even as he minimizes differences between the past and the present. Reading ancient and modern history, he maintains, "we are continually struck with the analogy which exists between the epidemic diseases signalized by the general name of PLAGUE, and which decimated all the living beings, and those which more recently, and at the present moment, have startled the world by their fatal effects on men and animals" (18). Analogies, then, between human and animal plagues structure his arguments for a comparative pathology based on a single principle: there are timeless "physiological and pathological laws which rule and determine the phenomena of organic matter, whether in health or sickness" that have been set forth in the Bible (19). Paraphrasing Christ's words to the apostles at the Last Supper, Bourguignon emphasizes the status of cattle as sacrificial animals within Christian agrotheology.

Central to the "wealth and happiness" of man, he continues, is a divinely sanctioned meat-based diet. "We are the sovereign masters of animals," he declaims, and "their lives must be given to preserve our own; but on their well-being and happiness our own well-being and happiness also depend" (204). This relationship of beneficent interdependence, however, is undermined by the common practice of butchers selling infected meat, a failure of scientific understanding, moral and socioeconomic responsibility and sound public health. Were tainted meat to compromise the health of Britons, they would more easily fall prey to diseases, such as cholera; and if cholera should reach the shores of England at this critical conjuncture,

> it will find organisms most ready to receive its virus. Then, indeed, if the typhic miasma come to mix and blend with the choleraic miasma, all living beings will have to contend with the most deleterious causes of alternations in their health, and we may (God send it be otherwise!) witness one of those measureless calamities which, known in the former ages as the *Black Pestilence*, decimated cattle and men indiscriminately, and which, when we read the sorrowful accounts of it in history, make the flesh creep with affright. (181)

In Bourguignon's apocalyptic scenario, typhus and cholera may not be zoonotic, but they are pathologically interdependent; together they can lead to horrors somewhere between the biblical plagues of Egypt and Mary Shelley's *The Last Man*. His historical analogy to "the *Black Pestilence*" underscores the ways that nineteenth-century health regimens remain enfolded within still-vibrant ideas of agrotheology. Despite his distaste for blanket slaughter policies, and despite his claim that, like sick men, cattle "must be treated," ultimately Bourguignon admits that he will "tolerate" a cost-benefit analysis that demonstrates the "painful necessity" of killing "diseased animals" (205). Without targeted culling, cattle "will return to us the sufferings and diseases of which they die a hundred times over" (204). Traditional quarantine and culling policies advocated in the eighteenth century seemingly become a last resort for a nineteenth-century medical system alert to the consequences of zoonotic spread.

In this respect, Bourguignon, like Leonard Mascall centuries earlier, chastises those in the cattle business for mere profit-taking, and, again like Mascall, bases his critique on a pastoral politics grounded in agrotheology. Bourguignon asserts that the "same great measures which are known to maintain and restore the health of human beings will also maintain and restore the health of cattle" (272). This ethos of shared susceptibility and shared biophysical response to hygienic improvements allows Bourguignon to moralize about the conditions of the nineteenth-century international livestock trade by emphasizing similarities, and his text contains touching accounts of the internal lives of cows and the humans who care for them.

In explaining the dangers of driving cattle long distances, for example, Bourguignon describes their plight in the language of nineteenth-century sentiment: Under ideal conditions, "their calm, monotonous life," he claims, "has been as regular as the course of time; . . . they are all gifted with a nervous sensibility of which the vulgar have no notion" (100). These are not the cattle being fattened in early modern Venice or herded across the steppes, but the idealized beings of seventeenth- and eighteenth-century landscape painting. Those cattle "reared and fed beneath the domestic thatch," he claims, "were grateful for the care they had received; their master was endeared to them, they would run to meet his coming, answer to their name, and lick his hand with fondness" (101). Here English cows hover between being livestock and domestic pets capable of demonstrating recognizeable emotions: gratitude, recognition, even love ("fondness"). In some ways, the cows embody a paternalistic vision of happy peasants, grateful for what they receive. "In contrast," he continues, those cattle imported from Russia, "half-fed and athirst,"

> are forced to make long journeys afoot; or since the construction of railways, to be heaped together confusedly in a locomotive pen. There, the shaking, the sudden starts, the friction of five hundred wheels on the rails, the horrid snorting of the engines, alarm and terrify them to such a degree as to turn the whole mass of their blood. (102)

In ways that recall abolitionist accounts of the Middle Passage, Bourguignon invokes not only the "torture" of animals going nine or ten days without nourishment, but the psychological terrors of transportation. Their health deteriorates, and they arrive in a "state of general derangement and disease" (103). Their suffering serves as a moral and scientific indictment of the international cattle trade and the commodification of sentient beings.

Even worse, once in London, the Russian cows, packed into densely populated market stalls, infect the air of the metropolis, before finally reaching the "manorial farms of the wealthy patricians" (121). Even on these "plots of rural ground" where "men... thought the genius of epizootia would not invade" (121), the cattle die painful and, at least, partly avoidable deaths. While admitting that some healthy and well-treated cattle will succumb to the plague, Bourguignon drives home the analogy to cholera:

> as the cholera chiefly fixes itself upon the sickly, the ill-fed, the unclean, upon those who live in crowded dwellings and badly ventilated rooms; so, too, does the typhus choose its victims among the stalls and stables of those graziers who keep their cows tied up for years to the rack, giving them neither air nor exercise, and feeding them, not on that diet which their health requires, but on those things which add to their milk and increase their flesh. (289)

His critique of Victorian practices foreshadows the principles of factory farming: zeal for profit threatens the health of animals and humans alike. To restore the health of Europe's herds, he calls on farmers to stop selling diseased flesh (297); separate sick and sound cattle, putting both on a moderate diet and a strengthening tonic (299); and clean and fumigate their stalls (301). Because weak cattle succumb to rinderpest in the same way that weak people succumb to cholera, he contends, people who eat infected meat are likely to fall victim to the cholera outbreak knocking at Europe's door. In this agrotheological fever dream, farmers and butchers, rather than physicians and veterinarians, are the last checkpoint between droves of diseased cattle and a multi-species plague scenario that "make[s] the flesh creep with affright."

Playfair, 1745, and the Cattle Diseases Prevention Act

After considerable debate, Parliament passed the *Cattle Diseases Prevention Act 1866;* it restricted imports and transportation of cattle across Britain, required the culling of sick cows (with compensation), and—in line with sanitary principles developed during cholera outbreaks—advocated "hygienic measures which experience acquired in other diseases shows to be important in the spreading of contagion, and in diminishing the intensity of its attack."[8] Lyon Playfair—British chemist, Liberal member of Parliament, sanitary movement advocate, and one of the authors of the act—elaborates on the reasoning behind this legislation in his text *The Cattle Plague in its Relation to Past Epidemics and to the Present Attack* (1866). He acknowledges "this disease is of foreign importation," but attributes its rapid growth and spread "to our gross neglect of sanitary laws as regards our cattle" (58). Russia is either the "birthplace" of cattle plague "or its nursery" (18) in part because, at any given time, the Czar's realm is breeding about eight million cattle. During the "good season," merchants buy the cattle, healthy and diseased, and move them to fairs in Hungary (58). As the plague "penetrates Western Europe," it becomes increasingly virulent: on the steppes, the plague may carry off half the cattle, and in Hungary the mortality rate rises to about 65%, but on its first appearance in England it kills "upwards of 90 per cent" (26). These grim statistics inform Playfair's belief (harking back to Layard almost a century earlier) that cattle plague is more akin to smallpox than to cholera, typhus, or any other disease and that therefore rinderpest eventually may respond to effective vaccines. But given conditions in 1866, when there is no cure for cattle disease, the government has no choice but to return—and return quickly—to a version of the regulations adopted during Britain's last outbreak in the 1740s and 1750s.

Playfair's historical argument, significantly, focuses on resemblances, not differences, between 1745 and 1865; dismissing any possibility of curing stricken cattle, he combines pastoral politics with plague bureaucracies, subjecting farmers to the demands of an international food system and its interventionist medical regime. As in Bourguignon's treatise, analogies between human and animal diseases are central to his argument. "It is curious," he writes, "to read *The Gentleman's Magazine* from 1745 to 1757, and see how history repeats itself":

> the same energetic correspondents who now send their lucubrations to the newspapers, protesting against the use of the pole-axe, advocating or opposing the system of compensation for slaughtered cattle, framing insurance societies, fighting against ideas of contagion, and importation of the disease, and describing all kinds of cure. We have not yet seen one method of cure,

[8] I quote this section of the report from Playfair's extended defense, in *Cattle Plague* (1866), 61.

> except homoeopathy, tried in 1865, which was not tried and found wanting in the plague of 1745. (15)

This lack of progress is vexing because in 1866 England is embedded in a more highly developed network of international markets and transportation systems (steamships, railways), and the nation is even more exposed to the ravages of cattle plague: "The density of her population, the large quantity of her horned stock, and, above all, the enormous facility of communication by railroad, make her peculiarly liable to the ravages of a contagious disorder, and render the prospect of eradicating it, within any reasonable time, either by slaughter or by curative and disinfecting measures, almost hopeless" (45). Playfair's use of the phrase "almost hopeless" is telling. It explains the frustration we saw in the *Punch* cartoon: while experts argue, cattle and their owners suffer. Playfair disagrees with the "minority" of those writing the Commission report, who wanted to resurrect the measures pursued between 1745 and 1757, which were even then "found signally inoperative" (46). Yet as a member of Parliament, he blames people in the cattle industry as well as the government for the consequences of the current outbreak. Despite all the grumbling about government "interference" in 1745, the people ended up regretting "most bitterly" (46) that they did not follow official recommendations for quarantining and culling. In Playfair's mind, then, 1745 becomes a cautionary tale about non-compliance and spotty enforcement of regulations, a vicious cycle dragging on for twelve years while the disease erupted, receded, and erupted again.

A century later, the industrialized market has intensified and no pasture or market is safe. Bourguignon asserts that "the markets of this immeasurable London have for many years been supplied with horned cattle from every country: from France, Holland, Belgium, Podolia, Poland, Prussia, Austria, Hungary, and Russia" (110). Playfair, like others, zeroes in on this trade, advocating a "total stoppage of movement of cattle," despite objections that such drastic measures are premature and despite protests "against this despotic interference with business and traffic" (47). But his idea of a "total stoppage" is this: rather than driving cattle from the steppes to Hungary, then transporting them from Hungary to England to be fattened, cattle should be fattened and slaughtered closer to their grazing pastures on the steppes. Shipping "dead meat" rather than live cattle "must be begun at once, for it is only in cold weather that we can get a sufficient supply of dead meat from abroad to aid us in our deficiencies at home" (48). While this solution wipes out middlemen in the cattle trade, it promotes a new technology and a new industry: refrigerated railway cars ("reefers") to transport rendered cattle were being designed in the 1860s and were patented the following decade.

At some level, Playfair's reform efforts, his promotion of local sanitary interventions, and his hopes for a rinderpest vaccine, reflect his (and many of his contemporaries') sense of futility. "Preventative" measures in 1866 are almost invariably symptoms of scientific, environmental, and public policy failures. This insight strikes me as critical to understanding Playfair's contributions to cattle plague literature. In traditional histories of medicine, Playfair get characterized as a moderate contagionist, who tended to contextualize moral questions in terms of germ theory and environmental factors. He "denounced as 'fanatics' those who thought the cattle plague a punishment for whatever sins they most despised," writes Mark Harrison, "but believed that God had made laws governing creaturely welfare" and "that transgression of those would necessarily bring penalties" (Harrison 2013, 218). Like Bourguignon, Playfair argues that farmers—rather than doctors or veterinarians—should shoulder primary responsibility for mitigating the disease. Citing the Commission Report, Playfair, endorses their view that every farmer

> should look to the housing of his cattle in the present emergency, as he would to the housing of his own family, if cholera or other formidable disease were in his neighborhood. Through cleanliness of the houses, good drainage, freedom from evil smells, nourishing diet with pure air and water, cannot give immunity from the disease, but they may offer obstacles to its propagation. (61)

Mistreatment, Playfair argues, stems from farmers looking at cattle "in the double-light of flesh-making and manure-producing beasts"; even though this economic perspective is "right and natural," it is "neither natural nor right that the stalls in which the beasts are fed should be made the storehouse for this manure" (58). Conflating lessons learned about cholera, which can be spread through excrement, and bubonic plague, usually transmitted by fleas, he admonishes farmers that "if men herd among the manure voided by themselves, we know how soon pestilence would ravage them" (58), as it did in the fourteenth century by the Black Death. Extending this analogy, he claims that much as cattle "made glutton by their mode of fattening" become "prone to disease," "the upper classes in the thirteenth century," equally "gluttonous and unruly," fell to bubonic plague, "a scythe quite as keen for cutting down the well-conditioned members of society as it had used for the poorer classes" (59). If most people in the nineteenth century "no longer dread" the plague or its vectors of infection—"even in the porous cotton which comes to us from plague-infected Egypt"—it is not because medicine has developed an effective cure, but because sanitation has improved dramatically, at least for many of his readers, if not for the London poor.

The Cattle Plague in its Relation to Past Epidemics and to the Present Attack mentions cholera only four times, but the sanitary laws that Playfair hopes to establish for cattle are derived from the medical response to cholera, plague, and other human epidemics (Harrison 2013, 23, 33, 53, 61). These laws, significantly, turn on the analogy between humans and cattle, with which he ends his treatise. "The God of the human race," Playfair declares, "whose are the 'cattle on a thousand hills', governs this world by wise and beneficent laws, which are sufficient, when obeyed, to insure the wellbeing of his creatures" (62). The phrase "cattle on a thousand hills" comes from Psalm 50, which commends the Israelites for following divine laws; these include animal sacrifice, but the Psalmist reminds readers that, in contrast to the pagan gods, God does not *need* animal offerings: "For every beast of the forest *is* mine/ *And* the cattle on a thousand hills. / I know all the fowls of the mountains/ And the wild beasts of the fields *are* mine" (Psalm 50, verses 10, 11). Playfair reads the passage analogically, conflating men and beasts in ways that subsume the laws of sacrifice into physical law, or laws of nature: "The violation of these laws inflicts on us the penalties attached to their transgression"—notably, illness and suffering—"and it is our duty to discover, understand, and obey them" (62, n 46). In this context, similarities between human and animal disease engender a kind of cross-species empathy, especially apparent in Playfair's condemnation of the crowded, filthy railway cars essential to the international trade in livestock. Excoriating the poor treatment of animals during transport, he advocates for larger compartments with water troughs: "But such a simple device," he complains, "is much beyond the humanity of railway officials, who, as long as they can obtain cattle according to the present system of transport, choose to consider them as inanimate objects, to be treated with as little consideration as bales of merchandise" (61–62). As in the case of his contemporaries like Bourguignon, Playfair's advocacy for animal welfare is a by-product of an agrotheology that generated both the trade in animals and the diseases it is still trying to contain. The railway cars carrying live animals are part of a complex industrial system that must adapt to forestall the spread of rinderpest. New refrigeration cars can carry the carcasses of cattle slaughtered elsewhere, in the name of hygienic laws; their cargo no longer will need water troughs at all.

Pandemic Disinformation, Contagion, and Humanity

As the *Punch* cartoon indicates, debates about the best ways to counter the cattle plague found their way into the popular press, becoming stalking horses for larger sociopolitical and ideological positions. Even as veterinary professionals acted to support and extend the 1866 cattle bill, laypeople jumped into the debates with their own critiques and their own brands of disinformation. The most notable example was Henry Strickland Constable's *Observations Suggested by the Cattle Plague, about Witchcraft, Credulity, Superstition, Parliamentary Reform and Other Matters* (1866), a text that projected its ire about the bill onto the person of the veterinarian John Gamgee. Although Gamgee, unlike Playfair, was neither in Parliament nor on the Commission that produced and amended the acts, he was an outspoken and deeply political contagionist who, repeatedly, warned the British against the consumption of diseased animals and the unsanitary perils of free trade(Francis 430–31). After 1865, Gamgee delivered a series of public lectures in which he excoriated cattlemen, dairy farmers, and other "obstructionists" whose "selfishness and greed" (Spinage 236, n2) were on display during the current outbreak. In 1866, arguing on the side of contagionism and culling, he published a lengthy account of two international veterinary conferences devoted to cattle plague—1863 in Hamburg, 1865 in Vienna; his preface chastised the British government for ignoring his warnings and failing to act quickly when cattle disease appeared in July 1865 (Gamgee 1866). Strickland Constable mimics and misrepresents both the Cattle Plague Commission Report and Gamgee's "exceedingly entertaining" international proceedings: "I laughed . . . at the report of our own Commissioners on the Cattle Plague, in consequence of its inconclusiveness, want of unanimity and strong veterinary flavour, but it was the wisdom of Solomon in comparison with these German enunciations" (11). Spinage is no doubt correct that Strickland Constable's treatise "contributes nothing of value" to debates about the rinderpest outbreak, except to exemplify "the kind of perverse opinion Gamgee was confronted with, opinion held by educated and wealthy people" (235 n2). Yet Strickland Constable's know-nothing anti-contagionism remains significant for cultural historians and cross-disciplinary critics, especially for those who, 160 years later, are still battling the cherrypicking, omissions, and exaggerations of pandemic disinformation.

Like the treatise writers I have discussed, especially Bourguignon, Strickland Constable often compares rinderpest to cholera and accuses Gamgee of failing to see "the unity of principle between typhus in a man, and rinderpest in a cow, because he only has an eye for the differences" (48). But unlike these physicians, Strickland Constable is aggressively anti-contagionist, arguing that "the question of contagion or non contagion is . . . almost impossible to prove it one way or the other" (28). In his mind, the spontaneous generation of disease is a given, a position offering him a vantage point to ridicule all policies and strategies intended to confront every contagious disease. "In the newspapers printed in the winter of the year 1866," Strickland Constable writes,

> we read of a vast destruction amongst cattle, caused by poisonous influences which exist without beginning in, and flow without cessation from, some remote but unknown corner of the Russian deserts. We read of mysterious emanations that were carried by the winds for miles, and left death wherever they lighted. We read that this subtile power was conveyed by the birds of the air, by insects, by mice, by cats, by dogs, by rats; and that it was even carried and imparted by the very men who were appointed by the Government to prevent its spreading. (9)

His satire deploys the rhetoric of medieval and early modern mysticism—"influences," "emanations," "subtle powers"—that might have been lifted from an alchemical manuscript. Strickland Constable seizes on fundamental uncertainties to treat theories of contagion like witchcraft. In one respect, he turns the rhetoric of scientific authority and truth-telling against itself. Because medical science cannot explain everything—a travesty of nineteenth-century claims for the value of the experimental method and progress in understanding epidemiology—for him it can explain nothing: no one "in the present state of science," he argues, can say why "one village is attacked and the next escapes,... any more than they can say in the case of cholera, or any other epidemic" (30). Without being able to identify causal agents, then, contagionists, like their superstitious and ill-informed ancestors, make up what he calls "idle theories," such as Jews poisoning wells or "subterranean vapours issuing from the clefts in the earth's surface," to account for the Black Death and for subsequent disease outbreaks among humans and livestock. His contemporaries' explanations for rinderpest as the product of "mysterious contagious emanations," (30) he asserts, ultimately derive from unconvincing attempts to hide their ignorance.

Through a series of pretended summaries mirroring *Punch*'s "The Essence of Parliament" (weekly and often humorous reports on Parliamentary discussion), Strickland Constable accuses the veterinarians at Gamgee's conferences of being self-interested quacks influenced by pre-modern pseudo-science and incapable of arriving at any consensus about how to manage the present plague, other than by mass culling. Partly by casting Gamgee and fellow scientists as "half-cultivated" (26) throwbacks to the eighteenth century and its plague bureaucracies, and partly by ignoring theories of contagion that do not fit neatly into a straightforward binary logic, Strickland Constable aligns himself—in ways that prefigure Health Secretary Kennedy and the MAHA movement—with a "modern" sanitary movement in which contagion does not figure at all. He claims that

> disease in cattle, if right notions prevailed, might in future be almost entirely prevented. My moral in all I have said, is, that good food, cleanliness, light, and open field management, would save us from a repetition of the disease for all time. The moral of Mr. Gamgee's book is, 'They are filthy, let them be filthy still;' for that all the diseases mentioned there in are inevitable dispensations of Providence. I preach food and air. Mr. Gamgee preaches slaughter. (53)

In such passages, Strickland Constable represents himself and his anti-contagionist, anti-regulatory views as humane, pious, and progressive—even identifying his position with Playfair's. Glossing over Playfair's contagionist beliefs by dismissing them as a "veterinary delusion," he recommends "the latter part of Dr. Lyon Playfair's little book about the Plague," which he then misrepresents. Playfair, according to Strickland Constable, says, "that the rapid growth of the disease, is owing to our gross neglect of sanitary laws; and that what is wanted, is by good management to make our animals proof against it as we have already done with men in the case of Oriental [bubonic] plague" (53). He seemingly has in mind Playfair's comparison between the Black Death infecting men "stalled like oxen on rush-covered floors" (Playfair 58) and rinderpest attacking cattle packed in manure-ridden stalls. But, as we have seen, Playfair never argued that "good management" makes animals immune to disease, only that such measures slow its spread. Moreover, he defined "contagious" explicitly, albeit in ways that Strickland Constable ignores or marginalizes: "there is a specific entity which causes the disease, and has the power of propagating its own species rapidly under favouring circumstances" (Playfair 23). By dismissing Playfair's clear statements on contagion even as he promotes Playfair's sanitary recommendations, Strickland Constable offers a master class in the rhetorical maneuvers of anti-scientific discourse—cloaking his prejudices in the mantle of common sense in order to market his book.

Strickland Constable's representation of his position as "modern" may seem jarring to twenty-first-century readers, but as Erwin Ackerknecht has argued, anti-contagionism peaked during the second half of the nineteenth century in the aftermath of Darwin's *Origin of the Species*. According to Ackerknecht, contagionism never was—and still isn't—"a mere theoretical or even medical problem" because it "found its material expression in the quarantines and their bureaucracy" (2009, 9).[9] Insofar as contagionism was associated with "old bureaucratic powers," such as the *cordon sanitaire*, Victorians who tried to reduce "state interference to a minimum" in the name of free trade found anti-contagionism—like anti-masking and anti-vaccination—both congenial and strategic; it allowed them to position themselves as reformers, "fighting for the freedom of the individual and commerce against the shackles of despotism and reaction" (Ackerknecht 2009, 9 n89). Clearly, Strickland Constable casts himself in this tradition. "A time may come," he pronounces, sarcastically, "when it will not be illegal for a man to cure his cow when she catches a cold" (37). He whines about a "tenant" who had forty animals infected "after the Act for the prevention of recovery had come into force," so [instead of being allowed to heal], "they were of course shot" (39). By the end of his treatise, he justifies his virulent attacks on economic grounds: "when I consider, that by their ignorant treatment, and blood-thirsty counsels, they have caused a loss to the community of a very great many thousand pounds, I do not think I have spoken too strongly" (54). In ways that may strike some readers as uncannily familiar, Strickland Constable represents a disdain for science and a defense of commercial interests as the ultimate form of patriotism. His calls for animal welfare cynically wave the tattered remnants of Christian pastoralism, even as he turns away from the dilemma of the fifth plague: that cattle suffer from diseases for which humans and their insatiable appetites are responsible.

[9] For a nuanced critique of anti-contagionism, see Hamlin (2009: 22–27).

Playfair's recognition of constitutional similarities between humans and animals helped lead him into progressive social causes, including sponsorship of the second version of the 1876 Cruelty to Animals Act, the so-called Vivisection Act, which required the use of anesthesia on vertebrate experimental subjects. Even in the midst of a global zoonotic pandemic, animal welfare concerns glimmer in his complaint about "filthy" stalls; one hears echoes of Jeremy Bentham's lament that, thanks to ignorance and the biases of ancient philosophy, many animals "stand degraded into the class of things" (Bentham 1823, 2: 234–235). Strickland Constable, in contrast, is remembered now mostly for his eugenicist writings about race, and for manifestos with such titles as *Equality: A Socialist-radical Fallacy* (1897). His texts from the 1880s and 1890s invariably raise questions about the relationships between anti-contagionism and racist pseudoscience. In important ways, nineteenth-century anti-contagionism functions primarily as an act of negation, a rhetorical maneuver designed to shift the burden of proof onto scientists working at the forefront of germ theory. In the hands of Strickland Constable and other eugenicists, the belief that epidemics are inevitable slips too easily into the chilling position that epidemics are therefore a desirable means of population control. In the animal world, he claims, almost "the only natural evil is famine and its consequent diseases" (51). If food were plentiful, "animals would no longer have to work for their living," which would bring about "a state of things [...] so awful and destructive, that animal life would shortly cease to exist upon the globe. So with men, if they are not kept in some degree of order by plagues and diseases, following vice, dirt, and indolence, the race would soon become extinct" (51). For Strickland Constable, both cholera and rinderpest become litmus tests for healthy "races," or forms of natural selection. The origin and mode of transmission of these diseases is less important than their effects: to "cull" the human and animal worlds of their presumably inferior members. If he rejects the pole-axe on mercenary grounds, his rhetoric favors a society in which food and hygiene, rather than medicine, determine the health of the social body. And because food and hygiene depend, in large measure, on imperial wealth and the exercise of imperial and colonial power, these socioeconomic inequalities determine who will be exposed to, treated, and consequently better positioned to survive a global pandemic.

"The Nasty Coat"

Throughout this study, we have seen that the medicopolitical and religious literature of cattle disease has been *eruptive*—it proliferates in response to immediate crises, generates often heated debates, then slows to a trickle when cattle plague does not seem to be an immediate threat. In this respect, it follows patterns we recognize from the literature of the bubonic plague or, for that matter, from the literatures of the AIDS epidemic and the COVID pandemic. The same patterns might be said to hold true for literary texts: *De Mortibus Boum* was republished periodically in response to, or in anticipation of, devastating outbreaks among livestock; bovine elegies appear as campy tributes to sensibility and invitations to animal welfare; the threat of potential disease hovers over more canonical works like Defoe's *Farther Adventures* and James Thomson's *The Seasons*. The 1866 plague served as the basis for at least one novel tackling rinderpest outbreaks head on, Sophie Amelia Prosser's *The Days of the Cattle Plague* (1872). Prosser (1807–82), neé Dibdin, was the granddaughter of the eighteenth-century songwriter and occasional playwright, Charles Dibdin, and married to a surgeon turned clergyman. Beginning in 1867, when she was 60, she began publishing novels and collections of tales with the Religious Tract Society. Among her many publications during her fifteen-year career was the only English novel to take the cattle plague as its narrative focus; the plot, to some extent, hinges on Victorian plague bureaucracies, and examines, with agrotheological specificity, the consequences of the 1866 outbreak for humans and animals.

Written six years after the 1866 epizootic, *The Days of the Cattle Plague* begins with a substantial, well-researched preface about the history of contagious cattle disease, justifying the government's policy during previous outbreaks. Prosser refers to the 1714 epizootic, Thomas Bates's recommendations (discussed in Chap. 4), and the presence of an "extreme drought" (8); the 1745–46 plague; and the "more destructive outbreak" (9) of 1866. Like Playfair and other contemporaries, she recognizes that the most recent epizootic has been "more destructive" because improved methods of agriculture have resulted in larger herds. From the census reported in "daily papers," Prosser calculates that by March of 1866, of Great Britain's 4,935,641 cattle, 253,723 had been "attacked," 149,805 had succumbed, and 52,411 had been slaughtered to prevent further spread—an "immense number" of these slaughtered cattle had been "butchered and sold at a heavy sacrifice as inferior meat" (10). Even though "much ridicule was excited by what was deemed a needless and foolish excess of precaution" in the government's stamping out policy, she argues that "it was justified by the result" (13). To cement her case, Prosser argues that the "absolute isolation" of parishes such as Hodnet and Woollerton kept outbreaks there from spreading.

Six years after these measures went into effect, Prosser continues, Great Britain faces another crisis in the making. *The Days of the Cattle Plague* went to press in October 1872 when, she argues, "we are threatened with a fresh outbreak of the pestilence" (13). She recounts a newspaper article about an infected farm at Yapham, in Yorkshire, "the centre of a splendid agricultural district" (13). After one beast died and another fell ill, a veterinary surgeon, the cattle inspector for the district, identified the disease as rinderpest, and ordered the entire herd of 22 to be shot and buried. A *cordon sanitaire* of one mile around the field was "proscribed": no persons or animal could be removed or brought into the district; the footpath across the field "was stopped"; and "all dogs were ordered to be destroyed" (14). The Privy Council subsequently prohibited markets, fairs, sale, and exhibitions of cattle within the city of York and its surrounding boroughs. Movement of cattle from the region was halted, except by special license from the local authority. In marked contrast to Strickland Constable and other critics of quarantine and cull policies, Prosser introduces her novel by supporting both the principle of contagion and efforts to contain rinderpest through a combination of science and prayer: "it is hoped that, by the blessing of God," she ends the preface, "these prompt and decisive measures will prove efficacious to preserve us from a recurrence of this dreaded calamity" (14). In this respect, Prosser's novel exhibits a late nineteenth-century version of agrotheology, based on the compatibility of divine protection and up-to-date medical, socioeconomic, and veterinary practices.

The novel itself focuses on a dairy farming community somewhere south of Cheshire, introducing the inhabitants of Godsham, one of the first farms struck by rinderpest. The epizootic follows a significant drought. The Flints, a comparatively well-to-do but imperfect couple, are long-term tenants of Godsham—he is given to drink, and she to class insecurity, racist fears, and self-righteous vanity. Their ward, the deeply religious Nicholas Scores (not surprisingly in a novel published by The Religious Tract Society), is the grandson of their landlord, Gabriel Scores, the "largest landed proprietor in the district" (26). After marrying a "dairy girl," Nicholas's father, disowned by the outraged Gabriel, died of a "low fever" in poverty; Nicholas's mother perished soon thereafter. The orphaned Nicholas fell to the care of local charity until, shamed by his neighbors, Gabriel grudgingly offered a small allowance to the Flints to house "the brat," if only to spare the parish the expense of raising him. Now twenty and known for being both "patient and submissive" (27), Nicholas does chores for the Flints, but also travels the region around Godsham passing out religious tracts, hoping to make converts. The reader encounters other residents of the county at a religious meeting devoted, in part, to finding missionaries to travel to New Zealand. Mrs. Flint attends this meeting, but repeatedly falls asleep, only to be jerked awake by the words "cattle plague." "What!" she thinks, alarmed: "A disease abroad that struck down whole droves in just a few hours—that made the rich poor, that made the affluent beggars, in a few days!" (63). Of course, this is precisely what happens to the Flints. Within "a few days," rinderpest hits their farm and devastates their herds; unable to pay rent, they appeal to Gabriel Scores, who turns them out, callously advising them to emigrate. Their neighbors the Gunsbury's, however, reach out in Christian compassion to rescue the aging couple, offering them a temporary place at Broad Oak until they can make other arrangements. The Gunsburys's daughter Patty (who is in love with Nicholas) even purchases and returns some of Mrs. Flint's most meaningful pieces of furniture when the house goods go to auction.

Despite the moral shortcomings of some of the landowners, like Gabriel, and the socially ambitious Flints, *The Days of the Cattle Plague* is clear in its defense of farmers during the 1866 outbreak. According to her calculations, Prosser declares that the loss across affected regions was "fully four million pounds sterling"—a "pecuniary disaster" which, "among any other class, except our placid and enduring agriculturalists," would have "created a panic" (10). With exception of the hard-hearted Gabriel, who resists joining other large landowners in supporting a fund for stricken farms like Godsham—"I have very little stock…Corn land now chiefly, and I'm insured"—the farmers (and even the Flints, eventually) submit themselves to God's will and government policy. Medical science and Christian compassion reinforce the values embodied in placid and enduring agriculturists. Prosser is careful to defend farmers against accusations of poor husbandry, staple accusations of the sanitary movement. Patty, for one, relieves farmers of responsibility for diseases that resist the best efforts of both veterinary science and prayer. "This isn't like anything else, you mind," she declares, "We've had lung-disease, and fall-foot, and slobber mouth, and all manner, and they don't always turn out well; but there's some hope of managing them. This!—You may as try to manage the arrow up in the sky. Goodbye to it, and let it take its way,—it will, let it or not" (143). Patty's catalogue of common diseases is intended to reinforce the *impossibility* of managing rinderpest medically: "Lung-disease" may be caused by a variety of pathogens (viral, bacterial, parasitic, fungal); fall-foot may either be bacterial foot rot or viral foot and mouth disease; slobber mouth is likely slaframine poisoning, caused by forage contaminated by fungus. Abraham, an amiable local poet and balladeer, similarly describes the progress of rinderpest as inevitable: "We shall go like links in a chain; it's just the same as a match to a powder train—there's no stopping it" (85). Cattle plague remains, for Prosser, as it does for writers in previous centuries, an evil to be feared, contained, and endured.

Since Susan Sontag, we are alert to the ways that human illness functions as a metaphor (Sontag 1978). This is no less true of cattle plague, whose transmission, as we have seen in previous chapters, has been described as a "bane upgathering" (Lucretius), "a scourge" (Bible), a "Universal Blow" (Virgil), a "dire creeping" (St. Severus), a "taint" (Shakespeare), "a pestilential heat" (Dryden), "a poison" (Lancisi), and "a corruption" (Defoe). For Prosser, however, rinderpest is a material rather than metaphoric plague, and she does not take the traditional path of seeing outbreaks as evidence of divine displeasure. Unlike her contemporaries, who tend to reason analogically in searching for similarities between rinderpest and human diseases, especially smallpox and cholera, Prosser focuses almost exclusively on the inevitable "chain" of transmission and the refusal of the farmers to panic. In a tour of the Gunsburys's farm, Mr. Flint dons a work coat that his wife had sent over from the now-abandoned Godsham. Millie, the Gunsburys's granddaughter, goes "pale" when Flint carelessly picks her up on a ramble across the farm; she then reports her horror to her Aunt Patty on their return: "what a bad coat that man wears—nasty coat!" (149). In brief, the "rough brown" coat was infected with rinderpest; even though Mrs. Flint had had it "bacca'd," or fumigated with tobacco, a cow they visited in the morning was taken ill with the plague that night. The chain of transmission takes its grim course: "it spread as it had done at Godsham, till Broad Oak had become a scene of equal desolation" (150). Rather than blame the Flints, the Gunsburys double down on their piety: "Let us ask God's blessing on what he has provided; from day to day we must receive our bread at his hands" (150).

Shortly thereafter, in answer to this prayer, Nicholas, who had planned to emigrate to Prince Edward Island, returns from London with news that his grandfather Gabriel has died without leaving a will. Consequently, he inherits a large enough fortune to marry Patty, who moves with Millie and her recently widowed grandfather to Park End, the family estate. At the novel's conclusion, Nicholas sends the chastened and spiritually improved Flints back to Godsham, with a promise to re-stock their herds and to return to the financial and moral security of a "placid" agricultural life.

In some ways, *The Days of the Cattle Plague* returns to the agrotheological principles of *De Mortibus Boum*, written centuries earlier: wealth resides in stock; livestock are vulnerable ("so quick a path there is for evil things!"); compassion is a virtue ("A shared burden becomes less heavy"); plague trumps good husbandry; and resigning oneself to the divine will, followed by a spiritual reawakening, can lead back to earthly wealth ("simple purification of the soul enjoys the hoped for good things"). One could even argue that, in Prosser's region of dairy farms and farmers somewhere south of Cheshire, as in *De Mortibus Boum*, human community turns out to be an *effect* of infection. The movement of cattle stops, and, in that standstill, two characters find love, another humility, another sobriety, and several Christian fortitude. But *The Days of the Cattle Plague* was written in the context of a highly developed plague bureaucracy whose injunctions, for Prosser, need to be defended in the face of those landowners, financiers, and middlemen, like Strickland Constable, who fear the loss of profit and free trade more than they do pandemic disease. In this respect, the novel counters what Foucault calls "state-phobia," the belief that the state inevitably tries to extend its authority over every aspect of existence, by offering narrative examples of how contagion spreads and how to stop its progress (Dean and Villadsen 2016). Mr. Flint's "nasty coat" is critical to this process. If wearing "rough brown" is an unfortunate sign of the oft-drunken farmer's overall carelessness, it is also an opportunity for the Gunsburys, now ruined, to share in and alleviate their neighbors' suffering. If it is a call for isolating communities when disease has been discovered, it is also a recognition that all boundaries are porous.

At the missionary meeting in *The Days of the Cattle Plague*, before rinderpest devastates the farms and estates, several women mention plague in "Rupert's Land" (British territory in Canada), "South India," and "West Africa" (65). "I had no idea," says one, "that the plague was so well defined, so sure, and so close" (65). Prosser, however, clearly did. By 1871, railroads and steam powered ships enabled the shipment of live cattle "in numbers," writes Gordon Scott, "previously impossible" (Scott

2000, 15). The year before the publication of Prosser's novel, in 1871, an important report on cattle plague in India was released.[10] The Commission had been formed in 1869 to study "the numerous outbreaks of disease which have of late years occurred in India"—losses in the hundreds of thousands. The Commission concluded that murrain may be attributed to "increasing civilization" in India, by which they mean jungle clearing, road building, "extending agriculture," "buying and selling" with other parts, all of which "provides greater facility for the spread of contagious diseases of stock" (*Report* vi). What the Commission calls "increasing civilization" we might call "agrilogistics," with its own epidemic feedback loops. Calcutta, for example, already offered in 1869 a case study in the "evil effect of crowding" livestock, and an example of how the "increasing demand of animals for slaughter"—that is, for table meat—had altered their status: whereas cattle once held status as "a representative of means or wealth," they were now "an agency of wealth," products in a meat market. Their losses by murrain, paradoxically, both "attract more attention" and more need for "repressive measures" (*Report* viii). By "repressive measures" the Commission means the kind of surveillance and mitigation bureaucracies that, as we have seen throughout these chapters, force cattle into a medico-economic network that includes, without being limited to, veterinary medicine. As the Commission puts it, the price of stock has risen, so that "the need of adopting measure to protect against loss is more urgent now, and yearly becoming more so" (xviii).

After India, cattle disease spread to Southeast Asia and then to Africa. White traders had already introduced contagious bovine pleuropneumonia to South Africa, which had killed 50% of the cattle in the Zulu Kingdom (Ballard 1986: 421–450). In 1887, infected Indian cattle, imported by Italians to "supply their campaign against Somalia," became established in the Horn then moved throughout South Africa—a vast region already suffering from European cholera. As Pule Phoofolo writes,

> What made the rinderpest crises even more ominous than European cholera, and loaded it with explosive social and political potential, was the nature of the disease. While cholera attacked people, who died and left their property behind, the rinderpest spared the people to watch with utter shock and suspicion as their most valued means of livelihood perished dramatically. (1993: 114)

[10] *Report of the Commissioners Appointed to Inquire in to the Origin, Nature, etc. of Indian Cattle Diseases* See also Mishra (2011a, 2011b, 587–619; 2011c: 317–38).

Because cattle provided milk, meat, tractive power, clothing, fuel, and fertilizer, "utter shock" had devastating socioeconomic consequences. Between 1896 and 1898, rinderpest killed over 95% of South African herds, which resulted in the collapse of the ox-wagon transport system; at the same time, several years of drought and inflated food prices brought on human disease outbreaks, some of them caused by eating badly prepared meat from cattle that had died of the rinderpest. "Suspicion" was rampant because it was widely believed that white men had poisoned the cattle in order to coerce Africans into service (Phoofolo 119). European missionaries, "especially those of Protestant stock," hailed the outbreak as a "godsend" that could teach indigenous Africans a lesson: "by the sweat of your brow shall you live." This sentiment, widely circulated by such newspapers as the *Christian Express* (May 1, 1897), represented plague as a divine catalyst that could drive "native labor from the fields into the mines, the stores, the railways, and the wharves" (cited in Phoofolo 139). Rinderpest, as Phoofolo demonstrates, gave cover for the colonial state to extend its hegemony through mitigation and containment measures, including forced sanitary measures, new border guards, and land grabs. Unfenced African cattle lands were confiscated and modified for the sake of instituting European agricultural practices.

The exploitative effects of government plague bureaucracies and colonial missionaries in India and Africa are outside the scope of this book. I end here, however, in order to emphasize a point about plague bureaucracies. "To be successful," writes Prosser about the Privy Council's mitigation orders, "the isolation" must "be absolute" (11). If Flint's "nasty coat," attests to the impossibility of *absolute* isolation and *absolute* immunity, so do the horrific Indian and African rinderpest outbreaks. "Absolute immunity," then, is perhaps the most deceiving and dangerous metaphor of all, in part because it denies the epidemic feedback loop of a grain-and-cattle-based culture in which Godsham and Great Britain and, by this time, much of the rest of the world had become entangled. Plague bureaucracies have differential effects—not simply on cattle, who were regularly put to death and shoved into mass graves—but also on the populations who occupy and sometimes defend their vastly different positions within the sprawling agrotheological-medical complex. To explore our collective, if differential, capture within the epidemic feedback loops of agrotheology—to engage in a medical posthumanities—is not to ignore the human for the sake of the nonhuman animal, but to insist on our historical reality as living beings among other living beings, all of us vulnerable to fear, hunger, contagion, hope, and cure.

References

Ackerknecht, Erwin H. 2009. Anticontagionism between 1821 and 1867. *International Journal of Epidemiology* 38 (1): 7–21.

Anonymous. 1866. *The Human Blight and Cattle Blight, or an Explanation of the Cholera and Cattle Plague*. London: Longmans and Green.

Arnold, David. 1986. Cholera and Colonialism in British India. *Past and Present* 113:118–151.

Atkinson, Lucy Sherrard. 1863. *Recollections of Tartar Steppes and Their Inhabitants*. London: John Murray.

Ballard, Charles. 1986. The Repercussions of Rinderpest: Cattle Plague and Peasant Decline in Colonial Natal. *The International Journal of African Historical Studies* 19 (3): 421–450.

Bashford, Alison. 2003. *Imperial Hygiene: A Critical History of Colonialism, Nationalism, and Public Health*. London: Palgrave Macmillan.

Bentham, Jeremy. 1823. *An Introduction to the Principles of Morals and Legislation*. London: W. Pickering.

Bourguignon, Honoré. 1869. *On the Cattle Plague: or, Contagious Typhus in Horned Cattle. Its History, Origin, Description, and Treatment*. London: Churchill & Sons.

British Medical Journal. 1866. 2 (301): 388.

Budd, William. 1865a. The Siberian Cattle Plague; or, the Typhoid Fever of the Ox. *British Medical Journal* 2 (242): 169–179.

Budd, William. 1865b. *Memoranda on Asiatic Cholera, Its Mode of Spreading and Its Prevention*. Bristol: J. Wright.

Burney, Ian A. 2007. The Politics of Particularism: Medicalization and Medical Reform in Nineteenth-Century Britain. In *Medicine, Madness and Social History: Essays in Honour of Roy Porter*, ed. Roberta E. Bivins and John V. Pickstone, 46–57. Basingstoke: Palgrave.

Bynum, W. F. 1994. *Science and the Practice of Medicine in the Nineteenth Century*. Cambridge: Cambridge University Press.

Constable, Henry Strickland. 1866. *Observations Suggested by the Cattle Plague, about Witchcraft, Credulity, Superstition, Parliamentary Reform and Other Matters*. London: Dalton and Lucy.

Constable, Henry Strickland. 1888. *Ireland from One or Two Neglected Points of View*. London: Hatchards.

Constable, Henry Strickland. 1897. *Equality A Socialist-Radical Fallacy*. London: Liberty Review Publishing.

Cook, Gordon Charles. 2002. Thomas Southwood Smith FRCP (1788–1861): Leading Exponent of Diseases of Poverty and Pioneer of Sanitary Reform in the Mid-nineteenth Century. *Journal of Medical Biography* 10 (4): 194–205.

Davis, Mike. 2000. *Late Victorian Holocausts: El Niño Famines and the Making of the Third World*. London: Verso.

Dean, Mitchell, and Kaspar Villadsen. 2016. *State Phobia and Civil Society: The Political Legacy of Michel Foucault*. Stanford: Stanford University Press.

Delaporte, François. 1986. *Disease and Civilization: The Cholera in Paris, 1832*. Translated by Arthur Goldhammer. Cambridge, MA: MIT Press.

Evans, Richard. 1987. *Death in Hamburg: Society and Politics in the Cholera Years 1830–1910*. Oxford: Clarendon Press.

Fisher, J. R. 1980. The Economic Effects of Cattle Disease in Britain and its Containment, 1850–1900. *Agricultural History* 54:278–294.

Francis, John. 1962. John Gamgee (1831–1894): Our Greatest Veterinarian. *British Veterinary Journal* 118, 430–38.

Gamgee, John. 1866. *The Cattle Plague*. London: R. Hardwicke.

Gardner, James. 1865. Cholera. *The British Medical Journal* 2 (246): 282–284.

Gilbert, Pamela K. 2009. *Cholera and Nation: Doctoring the Social Body*. Albany: SUNY Press.

Hall, Sherwin A. 1962. The Cattle Plague of 1865. *Medical History* 6 (1): 45–58.

Hamlin, Christopher. 2009. Commentary: Ackerknecht and 'Anticontagionism': A Tale of Two Dichotomies. *International Journal of Epidemiology* 38 (1): 22–27.

Harrison, Mark. 2013. *Contagion: How Commerce Spread Disease*. New Haven: Yale University Press.

Hevia, James L. 2018. *Animal Labor and Colonial Welfare*. Chicago: University of Chicago Press.

Holt, Daniel M. D. 1856. The Pathology of Zymotic Diseases. *Boston Medical and Surgical Journal* 54 (19): 369–376.

Kolb, Raza. 2021. *Epidemic Empire: Colonialism, Contagionism, and Terror, 1817–2020*. Chicago: University of Chicago Press.

Layard, Peter. 1757. *An Essay on the Nature, Causes, and Cure of the Contagious Distemper among the Horned Cattle in These Kingdoms*. London: Printed for J. and F. Rivington.

Lindsay, William Lauder. 1857. The Cattle Murrain in Some of Its Aspects. *The Lancet* 69:496–499.

Mishra, Saurabh. 2011a. *Pilgrimage, Politics, and Pestilence: The Haj from the Indian Subcontinent, 1860–1920*. Oxford: Oxford University Press.

Mishra, Saurabh. 2011b. Beasts, Murrains, and the British Raj: Colonial Medicine in India from the Veterinary Medicine Perspective, 1860–1900. *Bulletin of History of Medicine* 85 (4): 587–619.

Mishra, Saurabh. 2011c. Of Poisoners, Tanners, and the British Raj: Redefining Chamar Identity in Colonial North India, 1850–90. *Indian Economic Social History Review* 48 (3): 317–338.

Muturi, Ephantus J., et al. 2019. Amylose Inclusion Complexes as Emulsifiers for Garlic and Asafoetida Essential Oils for Mosquito Control. *Insects* 10 (10): 337.

Otis, Laura. 1999. *Membranes: Metaphors of Invasion in Nineteenth Century Literature, Science, and Politics*. Baltimore: Johns Hopkins University Press.

Phoofolo, Pule. 1993. Epidemics and Revolutions: The Rinderpest Epidemic in Late Nineteenth-Century Southern Africa. *Past and Present* 138:112–143.

Playfair, Lyon. 1866. *The Cattle Plague in its Relation to Past Epidemics and to the Present Attack*. Edinburgh: Edmondston and Douglas.

Prosser, Sophie Amelia. 1872. *The Days of the Cattle Plague*. London: The Religious Tract Society.

Punch; or the London Charivari. 17 February 1866a.

Punch; or the London Charivari. 3 March 1866b.

Report of the Commissioners Appointed to Inquire into the Origin, Nature, etc. of Indian Cattle Diseases. 1871. Calcutta: Office of the Superintendent of Government.

Rosenberg, Charles E. 1962. *The Cholera Years: The United States in 1832, 1849, and 1866*. Chicago: University of Chicago Press.

Scott, Gordon R. 2000. The Murrain Now Known as Rinderpest. *Newsletter of the Tropical Agriculture Association* 20 (4): 14–16.

Servitje, Lorenzo. 2021. *Medicine is War: The Martial Metaphor in Victorian Literature and Culture*. Albany: SUNY Press.

Shuttleton, David. 2007. *Smallpox and the Literary Imagination, 1660–1821*. Cambridge: Cambridge University Press.

Smith, Thomas Southwood. 1866. *The Common Nature of Epidemics and Their Relation to Climate and Civilization*. Philadelphia: Lippincott.

Snowden, Frank M. 2019. *Epidemics and Society: From the Black Death to the Present*. New Haven: Yale University Press.

Sontag, Susan. 1978. *Illness as Metaphor*. New York: Farrar, Strauss, and Giroux.

Spinage, C. A. 2003. *Cattle Plague. A History*. Amsterdam: Kluwer Academic/Plenum.

Stepan, Nancy Leys. 1986. Race and Gender: The Role of Analogy in Science. *Isis* 77 (2): 261–277.

Tucker, James. 1860. *The Reformed Roman or Oriental Baths, Reviewed as Thermo-electrical Temples of Health: with Medical Remarks on the Nature and Scientific Treatment of Cattle Distempers by the Hot Air Bath*. Sligo/Dublin: Champion Office.

Tucker, James. 1865. *Essay on the Nature and Treatment of Cholera and Fever, With Medical Remarks on the Treatment of Cattle Plague*. London: Churchill & Sons.

Weisz, George. 2003. The Emergence of Medical Specialization in the Nineteenth Century. *Bulletin of the History of Medicine* 77:536–575.

Worboys, Michael. 1991. Germ Theories of Disease and British Veterinary Medicine. *Medical History* 35:308–327.

"Work on Cholera." 1866. *The Dublin Quarterly Journal of Medical Science* 42 (1866): 131–167.

Deadstock, a Coda by Lucinda Cole

What are the uses of elegy? To confirm that loss is real, that individual disappearance matters; that the rupture in the known world is pointed to, held up for attention, shared.

Mark Doty, "Can Poetry Console a Grieving Public?"

"Deadstock" refers to livestock who die as a byproduct of the live animal trade, to the billions of carcasses that, because of disease, accidents, and so-called natural losses, need to be removed, rendered, or otherwise vanished. Especially after the 2003 bovine spongiform encephalopathy outbreak, disposal became complicated in many places (Morehouse et al. 2021, 1). Rendering companies that previously hauled away deadstock for free now operated under government health regulations, and therefore instituted fees to offset costs; the common practice of leaving diseased carrion to scavengers in boneyards now presented significant ecological and health consequences. Carcasses were burned en masse. The trade in live animals has a gross production value in the trillions of dollars, and because livestock biomass has reached about 630 million tons, the problem of how to dispose of dead animals is, for livestock producers, almost as critical as the health of live ones. The sheer *scale* of the agricultural industry makes it almost impossible to imagine. When I first outlined *The Fifth Plague*, I imagined it—simply—as a kind of *Contagious* for cattle, an account of outbreak narratives and their real and imagined consequences, a

L. Cole, *The Fifth Plague*, Palgrave Studies in Animals and Literature, https://doi.org/10.1007/978-3-031-92793-5

bovine-centered history of pestilence (Wald 2008). I planned on including nineteenth-century rinderpest events in India and Africa, a project that still needs to be done. In my global, animal-centered ambition, I underestimated how cattle plague would draw science into its orbit, pushing farmers, physicians, and even kings into complex political maneuverings. Cattle themselves often disappear under discussions of scarcity, meat safety, and government overreach; more precisely, the machinery of agrilogistics forces actual animals into kind of ontological flux—sometimes a sentient being, sometimes a valued laborer, sometimes a mere commodity, but increasingly, the latter. There can be no cattle-centered history because these enormous numbers of live and dead cattle are by-products of an anthropocentric commercial and—in some sense, theological—enterprise driven by profit. My call for a medical posthumanities is forged in the face of these facts and motivated by a desire to chip away at an anthropocentric health humanities. A recent collection, *Keywords for Health Humanities*, contains an entry on "Pollution" along with scattered remarks about multispecies epidemics (thanks mostly to Christos Lynteris) but otherwise omits concepts such as "Zoonosis" and "Epizootic," categories that capture the interdependence of human and animal health.

As I have argued in this study, cattle plague itself is a subject on which most humanists—and especially most *literary* humanists—have an indifferent record. Rather than casting blame, though, I want to understand why. Obviously, British literature (much like the health humanities) is built on an aesthetic tradition governed by the production of human-centered affective relations, to which sick cattle are not easily accommodated. A sad and perhaps humorous example occurs in Prosser's *The Days of the Cattle Plague*, as the poet Abraham Barfoot, having composed and performed an impromptu "Ode to Liberty," is interrupted by the grumpy Gabriel Stokes, who wants to change the subject. Gabriel asks whether there is anything in the paper. "Yes," reads Barfoot, "'Direful Spread of the Rinderpest,'": "'Direful news, the herds of many are being swept away; few hope to escape; it is piteous to hear the groans of the poor cattle, and to see them dragged one after another to their graves in the deep-dug pit'" (Prosser 1872, 79). Gabriel relays the rest of the newspaper report, but the article turns his thoughts to poetry. "A good subject that for an ode. Wild animals are more picturesque than domestic ones; but 'the lowing herd,' that sounds tender" (79). Barfoot's distinction between the aesthetic qualities of wild animals and domestic ones hearkens back to Edmund Burke, who readily admits that the cries of "animals in pain and danger," especially "the angry tones of wild beasts," are "capable of creating great ideas," while carving out an exception for the "well known voice of some creature, on which we are used to look with contempt" (Burke 1757, 58). Are cattle included in Burke's carve out? Is Abraham Barfoot joking? Intentionally or not, "tender" captures the doubleness of cattle as both subject and object. "Tender" means "sensitively felt" or "delicacy of feeling," but also "easily masticated," "succulent"; moreover, it alludes to a form of currency, acknowledging the enduring relationship between cattle and wealth. In the novel, Barfoot, affectionately known as "Brum," is a good man. Gabriel wants to leave him the estate but, as a friend of Nicholas's father with a strong sense of justice, Barfoot ensures that Gabriel's intention to cut out his grandson from inheriting is never realized: Gabriel dies intestate, Nicholas inherits, and Mrs. Flint declares "Brum's a gentleman to the backbone" (175). Like Nicholas, Brum disdains greed. Yet in his desire to be literary, even he, it seems, cannot avoid minimizing the suffering of cattle or transforming it into a witticism. As animal, meat, and currency, cattle fit uneasily into any aesthetic category, their cries simultaneously both an opportunity for poetry and a dinner bell.

Or maybe Brum cannot stand to watch. Cattle plague treatises offer glimpses into the massive scale of individual suffering, a view otherwise made possible only by direct experience or by PETA videos, from which many people (myself included) quickly turn away. Among the most graphic of these treatises is Honoré Bourguignon's description of "about a dozen diseased" animals that the veterinary inspector had ordered removed to a "secluded fold near the slaughterhouses" for further medical inspection (Bourguignon 1869, 132). While most of the animals, "panting," "feverish," "dispirited," and "lean," "remained motionless where they stood," one cow "with a brisk and lively look, a quick open eye" watched them, he says, "with anxiety" (133). When it was her turn to be examined, she shook off the veterinary inspector; when others came to his assistance, "the fiery animal was suddenly seized by both horns, by the nostrils, and the tail," but still she "defended herself," shaking herself free (133). They backed her into the corner of the pen. She leapt over the bars, coming "down with all her weight upon her limbs, fracturing one of her forelegs." Her owner refused to believe she was diseased, so

> to convince him, she was driven off at once to the slaughter-house to be struck down; but, unfortunately, three or four others filled the required area, so that the poor cow was forced to witness the execution of her

> fellow-creatures before being killed herself. The look and posture of this cow, her excited yet terrified glance as she surveyed this scene of carnage, was one of those pictures which no pencil could draw; and although we acknowledge that man possesses an incontestable right to apply to his own use the dead or live matter of animals for his food and sustenance, we could not help feeling for the poor victim, slipping over the blood, and thus scenting death before receiving the stroke. (134)

Bourguignon, a medical man who witnessed hundreds of bleeding horses and scores of slaughtered oxen, describes himself as "not excessively sensitive," but the "affecting sight of that animal witnessing the slaughter of others and waiting her turn to die," he says, "touched us deeply" (135). In ways that anticipate Temple Grandin's calls for more friendly chutes on the way to slaughter, why, he asks, did men who pride themselves on compassion not at least "bandage the eyes of the doomed creatures [they were] going to sacrifice?" He calls on his readers to acknowledge how "these dumb animals we treat like inert matter" are sensitive and "conscious of pain"; we ought not to "forget that they are, like us, endowed with intelligence, so that when they are thus detained at the place of execution, all their senses and faculties being concentrated on their destroyer, they are fully conscious of the cruel fate which awaits them" (135). Within the massive infrastructure built around the livestock industry, the most humane actions become those of a death doula, allowing anxious animals a slightly less terrifying death.

Animal welfare policies—bandage their eyes, clean their stalls, lose the waving flags, give them bigger cages—nest within a livestock industry whose dirty secret Bourguignon expresses succinctly: cattle "will return to us the sufferings and diseases of which they die a hundred times over" (204). Calls for plant-based diets during animal plagues acknowledge that pathological interdependence between sick animals and humans. Robert Samber (Eugenius Philalethes), one of Defoe's contemporaries, writing in his 1721 *A Treatise of the Plague*, warns "that Men, if they would or could abstain from eating the Flesh of Animals, wou'd find themselves much better in Health; for it is that dreadful mixture of the Souls, if I may say so, of so many thousand Animals, destroy'd to pamper one, that raises that terrible War in the Blood, which has made it a Prey to such Distempers, as have baffled the Skill of the most learned Physicians" (Philalethes 1721, 18). Samber's violent metaphor of a "War" in the "Blood" caused by scores of animals "destroy'd to pamper one" comes close to contemporary animal rights discourse, even as his appeal is grounded in anxieties about human health. Indeed, the two, already entwined in pastoral politics, quickly transition during major epizootic events into the risk regulation policies of what Foucault calls governmentality. "May the government," Bourguignon writes during a rinderpest outbreak, "which lavishes hundreds of millions upon the destructive engines of war, devote some portion of its ample means to the study of hereditary infections and contagious diseases! For these fatal epidemics decimate men as well as cattle, and we may at least ward off from our children the desolating disease which at present afflicts ourselves" (70). The One Health movement is, in many ways, a twenty-first-century response to the force of Bourguignon's plea. Insofar as it takes seriously the relationships among humans, animals, and the more-than-human world, One Health could be regarded as a scaled-up version of pastoral politics. Although, according to Abigail Woods, the focus of One Health has since its inception expanded beyond zoonotic diseases, most publications related to One Health appear in veterinary science journals. "These findings," she writes, "suggest that One Health is struggling to achieve its interdisciplinary aspirations, and that, in spite of its intention to advance health across all species, it is primarily humans that are benefiting" (2023, 27–28).

Can a medical posthumanities capture what is best about One Health, however imperfect—its multidisciplinary, non-anthropocentric ambition—in ways that open it up to those scholars and practitioners working in the health humanities? This remains an open question. In 2011, the United Nations held a ceremony to celebrate a vaccine for rinderpest, only the second time in history that medical science had eradicated a global disease. Yet, as Jeremy Youde notes, the long campaign to rid the world of rinderpest—unlike that to arrest smallpox—received "relatively little attention," probably because rinderpest does not infect humans. Compare this situation to writing about COVID-19. During and after the first years of the pandemic, the majority of humanists writing about COVID-19 have focused on the politics of human health and proper responses: masking, social distancing, vaccination, and the politics of politics. The problem identified by Roy Porter and reinforced by Abigail Woods, then, still stands, and is not exclusive to the history and philosophy of medicine: when most social scientists and humanists think of medicine and disease, they think of human medicine and disease (Woods et al. 2018, 12). Even in the midst of a global and zoonotic pandemic, even interdisciplinary scholars too often cast ourselves as the only players on the stage, a stage sometimes identified with Nature, with nonhumans consigned to the wings. The medical posthumanities may not solve this problem, but it at least offers a space of analysis. Neither a methodology nor a metaphysic, the medical posthumanities is an umbrella term for strategies and practices of affiliation through which the past, present, and future of multispecies "health" may be reimagined.

In concluding *The Fifth Plague*, though, I want to add a rider: in addition to being a space of analysis and a call to political action, the medical posthumanities, like the elegy, is a space of witnessing. Writing this book taught me that some problems seem so large and intractable, so difficult to transform, that we either displace them onto different and more manageable issues, or anesthetize ourselves to survive. Mark Doty, reflecting on the poetry produced immediately after 9/11, claims we "find ways to numb ourselves to the depictions of suffering"; maybe we learn to see pain as exotic, remote, repetitive, or aestheticized, "located within a beautiful pattern of shape and color, the eye arrested by the elegance of the photographer's vision" (2005). Or, as he puts it elsewhere, admitting that he has been unable to "coax climate change" into a poem, how does a poet address what "seems unredeemable?" (2006). Especially in the current global environmental, medical, and political chaos manufactured by Trump, Noem, Kennedy and a host of others, how do any of us? Can history actually help? With the exception of Jan Smit's iconic depiction of rinderpest in the Netherlands, the visual art I have discussed in this study projects mass animal die-off onto a neo-classical or Christian past. Most of the poetry, similarly, and especially what I have called "the bovine elegy" uses great mortalities as an invitation to individual spiritual awakening.

Yet the elegy, as Doty reminds us, however sentimental, also has a critical, affective purpose: "To confirm that loss is real, that individual disappearance matters; that the rupture in the known world is pointed to, held up for attention, shared" (2005). The death of cattle occurs on such a massive, quotidian, and largely invisible scale—in the United States alone, some 36 million every year—that it perhaps requires great plagues to bring into focus the animals, their diseases, and the unintended effects of the global industry that operates for profit at what Daniel Defoe calls a series "of circulating removes." Art, as Doty reminds us, "cannot be counted to mend the rifts within or without." Its work, instead, "is to take us to the brink of clarity" (2005). If a medical posthumanities offers nothing else, it can help us confront the suffering, theirs and ours, from which we are tempted to turn away. Although witnessing cannot solve the nested set of medical, ethical, and environmental problems we face, we can least meet them together, and more fully, than the health humanities so far have allowed.

References

Bourguignon, Honoré. 1869. *On the Cattle Plague: Or, Contagious Typhus in Horned Cattle. Its History, Origin, Description, and Treatment.* London: Churchill & Sons.

Burke, Edmund. 1757. *A Philosophical Inquiry into Our Ideas of the Sublime and Beautiful.* London: Printed for R. and J. Dodsley.

Doty, Mark, and Jane Hirshfield. 2020. The Worlds We Find Ourselves In: Mark Doty and Jane Hershfield in Conversation. *Guernica* (April 30, 2020). https://www.guernicamag.com/the-worlds-we-find-ourselves-in-mark-doty-and-jane-hirshfield-in-conversation/.

Doty, Mark. 2005. Return to Sender: Memory, Betrayal, and Memoir. *The Writer's Chronicle* 38.

Doty, Mark. 2006. Can Poetry Console a Grieving Public? *Poetry Foundation.* September 12. https://www.poetryfoundation.org/articles/68672/can-poetry-console-a-grieving-public-56d248475bff0.

Morehouse, Andrea T., Courtney Hughes, Nora Manners, Jeff Bectelli, and Jesse Tigner. 2021. Dealing with Deadstock: A Case Study of Carnivore Conflict Mitigation from Southwestern Alberta. *Frontiers in Conservation Science* 2: 1–13.

Morens, David, Edward Holmes, A. Sally Davis, and Jeffery K. Taubenberger. 2011. Global Rinderpest Eradication: Lessons Learned and Why Humans Should Celebrate Too. *Journal of Infectious Diseases* 204 (4): 502–505.

Philalethes, Eugenius [Robert Samber]. 1721. *A Treatise of the Plague.* London: Printed for James Samber.

Prosser, Sophie Amelia. 1872. *The Days of the Cattle Plague.* London: The Religious Tract Society.

Wald, Priscilla. 2008. *Contagious: Cultures, Carriers, and the Outbreak Narrative.* Durham: Duke University Press.

Woods, Abigail, Michael Bresalier, Angela Cassidy, and Rachel Mason Dentinger, eds. 2018. *Animals and the Shaping of Modern Medicine: One Health and Its Histories.* Basingstoke: Palgrave Macmillan.

Woods, Abigail. 2023. On Health: A 'More-than-Human History.' In *More Than-One-Health: Humans, Animals, and Environment Post-Covid*, ed. Irus Bravermen. London: Routledge, 27–40.

Youde, Jeremy. 2013. Cattle Scourge No More: The Eradication of Rinderpest and Its Lesson for Global Health. *Politics and the Life Sciences* 32: 43–57.

English Translation of *The Bucolic Song on the Deaths of Cattle* (*De Mortibus Boum*) by Michael Knierim

By Severus Endeleichus the Orator and Christian Poet,

with Notes by M. Johannes Weitzius
For
The magnificent and most noble man, Lord Jacques Bongars counselor of the most Christian king of France and magister of the court, etc.
At the end of the book is appended a copious index of words according to the sequence of lines.
Frankfurt
Egenolphus Emmelius, Book Printer
In the Year 1612

L. Cole, *The Fifth Plague*, Palgrave Studies in Animals and Literature, https://doi.org/10.1007/978-3-031-92793-5

Translator's Introduction to the Poem

The translation has been made from M. Johannes Weitzius's 1612 Frankfurt edition of the *Carmen Bucolicum*, printed by Egenolphus Emmelius. The public domain Latin text is readily available online, so no need was felt to present it again here. I have consulted J. A. Giles's 1838 London edition for clarification of occasional typographical errors in Weitzius's and Seber's notes.

The line numbers, chapter numbers, citations, etc. in the main text of the notes are by Weitzius or Seber. All footnotes are my own addition as well as any text in [brackets]. When there are major divergences between their numbering and modern editions, I have frequently added the modern numbers in the footnotes.

Throughout this document italics have been used to render Greek words and passages; all-capitals have been used to render German which reflects the large font used for it in the printed text. Latin has been rendered in normal fonts. Italics have also been used to render book titles.

When I was certain of the identity of a person, I have translated their Latin name into the more familiar vernacular version. In cases where I was not certain, I have left the Latin name unchanged.

Weitzius and Seber's notes well illustrate the commentators' vast learning and report many attitudes toward animals, illness, and empathy. However, a large number of their notes are purely concerned with defending and explaining the Latin of the author by providing numerous parallels

L. Cole, *The Fifth Plague*, Palgrave Studies in Animals and Literature, https://doi.org/10.1007/978-3-031-92793-5

from all periods of the language. These have been omitted as of little interest to those reading a translation, though the translator has not infrequently benefitted from their insights. Some passages on literary topoi and proverbs, while intelligible in translation, have been omitted as far from the subject of this volume. Of the theological passages some are directly relevant to animals and plagues while others are more remote from the topic, yet most of these have been included to help illustrate a vast cultural shift between the author of the poem and the early modern commentators which strikingly affects their attitudes toward the sacrality of animals as can clearly be seen in Seber's note on line 109 where the practice of signing cattle with the cross shocks him.

Michael Knierim
University of Illinios

Weitzius's Introduction

M. Johannes Weitzius, to the magnificent and most noble man, Lord Jacques Bongars counselor of the most Christian king of France and magister of the court, a most honorable patron.

Severus's bucolic poem has reached you, O most noble Bongars. Along with Seber "*the particular beloved of the nine muses,*"[1] I have begun to spend some hours on the work and to adorn it with notes as the need arose, chiefly at your instigation and *command*. For, to quote Theocritus, "*spring is not sweeter*"[2] than these dear verses which have first come before my eyes through your generosity which you show to all literary men and particularly to me.

It will be yours to judge whether I have achieved that aim for which you sent it to me. For if I pass your test, I will seem as if I am

> reclining at table in the midst of the stars
> with Jove, and stretching out my Trojan right hand to take
> the immortal (unmixed) wine.[3]

[1] Theocritus *Idyll* 11.6 in Gow's 1952 text. Theocritus addressed this complement to his learned doctor-poet friend, Nikias.

[2] *Idyll* 9.34.

[3] Statius, *Silvae* 4.2.10–2.

L. Cole, *The Fifth Plague*, Palgrave Studies in Animals and Literature, https://doi.org/10.1007/978-3-031-92793-5

And in return for your enviable liberality, humanity, and merits by which you deserve a world more literary than that of Europe, it is most fitting that the *assistant singers of the muses* give you an abundant return of "fame and benignant praise."[4] For you do not deem anything more beautiful than to exceed by virtue, glory, and merits those whom you excel in birth. Proceed joyfully, O great man, "and learn to deserve even more!"[5] *In this fragment* my zeal to please you will be manifest again and again. May God preserve and keep you for many many years as a fulcrum of the state and my patron O most magnificent Lord!

In Gotha,[6] MDCXI, St. Giles's Day,[7] on which (may Jehovah bid it be happy and joyful!) I turn 35 years of age.

[4] *Silvae* 5.3.250.
[5] *Silvae* 5.2.180.
[6] In Thuringia, Germany.
[7] September 1.

Beginning of the Song of Severus Endeleichus, the Orator: On the Deaths of Cattle

Characters: Aegon, Buculus, Tityrus.

Aegon: O Buculus, why is it that you wander alone groaning sadly with heavily downcast eyes? Why do your cheeks run with abundantly flowing tears? Let one who loves you know!

5. Buculus: Aegon, I beg you, let me bury my diseased senses in deep silence. For one who discloses misfortunes opens a wound. But one who covers it in silence closes it.
9. Aegon: The truth is the opposite of what you say, nor do you think rightly. For a shared burden becomes lighter, and whatever is covered boils down more violently. Conversation helps pain.
13. Buculus: Aegon, I was so wealthy in herds, that my cattle wandering along the rivers would even fill the hollows of the valleys, the plains and the ridges of the mountains.
17. Now all my hope in wealth has completely collapsed and the result of the long labor of all the seasons of my life has perished in two days. So quick is the path for evil things!
21. Aegon: There has been talk that this dire plague is already creeping upon us. It long ago devastated the Pannonians, Illyrians and Belgians too. And now, in its impious course, it seeks for us as well.

L. Cole, *The Fifth Plague*, Palgrave Studies in Animals and Literature, https://doi.org/10.1007/978-3-031-92793-5

25. But you, since you usually know how to drive away a dangerous death by healthful potions, why didn't you prevent it in advance with your healing hands?
29. Buculus: There are no obvious signs of this fearsome thing. The disease crushes whatever it takes hold of, nor does it allow its victim a period of weakness nor does it suffer any delays, but death comes before illness.
33. I had yoked a couple strong oxen to a cart. I had selected them with what skill I had. Their bells sang together, tinkling in harmony with their twin mind.
37. They were of the same age, their coats the same color. Both had the same tameness, the same strength, the same fate. For the pair collapsed in the middle of the furrow, conquered by the same death.
41. I was scattering seed grain[1] in the worked ground. The soil was friable with plenty of moisture. The plow had extended the furrows with ease. The ploughshare had never become stuck.
45. The left ox collapses in a sudden fit, the one that had been broken in last summer. I immediately unyoked his sad yoke-mate,[2] not fearing any more evils.
49. But, faster than I can say it, he followed in death, he who had always been healthy and sound. Then, shaking with long spasms in his flanks,[3] he laid down his conquered head.
53. Aegon: I am in pain, I am crucified, I mourn, I am in grief! My heart is consumed by your losses just as it is consumed by my own! But nevertheless, I think that your herds are safe.
57. Buculus: In my misery I was coming to that subject which weighs me down with sharper pain. For it would have been at least a very small consolation for the evil if future fertility were to give me that which the present plague had taken away.
61. But who would think it true that the offspring should perish at the same moment as well? I saw a young pregnant heifer sinking to the ground; I saw two souls perish in one body.

[1] or spelt.

[2] "coniunx" literally yoke-mate.

[3] "Ilia" means the area between the hips and the lowest ribs.

65. Here, refusing water, forgetful of grass, a young cow wanders with sinking tendons. Nor does she escape for long, but collapses heavily stumbling from the manacle of death.[4]
69. And on another side, a calf who had just been leaping and weaving playful paths went up to his mother and drew the plague from her diseased udder.
73. The mother was wounded with sorrow as she saw the hidden eyes of her calf and began lowing and groaning in misery. She sank down and wished to die.
77. Then, as if she feared that thirst would oppress his dry throat, dying she moved her udder to the dead one, there just where he lay. *Pietas* flourishes after death.[5]
81. Over here a bull, the husband and father of the solid herd with a strong neck and lofty, severe forehead is joyful as he pleases himself all too much. He collapses in the grassy meadow.
85. As many falling leaves are stripped from a forest when it is touched by the icy north wind; as many snowflakes as flow in fleecy clouds, so many were the deaths of kine.
89. Now all the ground is covered in corpses.[6] The bodies swell with bulging bellies. Their eyes whiten with bluish clouds. Their legs stiffen with tense feet.
93. Now columns of gloomy ill-omened birds continuously circle. Now the packs of dogs persist in enjoying the cattle's mangled viscera. Alas! Why don't they eat my own innards as well?
97. Aegon: Why is it? I ask, why is it that the sad fate of death has a varying measure and leaps past some while afflicting others? Look at that! Tityrus goes along happily with an intact herd!
101. Buculus: I am looking at it. Speak up Tityrus! What god snatched you out of these calamities so that the cattle plague that devastated your neighbors has not harmed you?
105. Tityrus: The sign, which they say is the cross of the only god worshiped in the big cities, Christ, the glory of the perpetual Divinity, and its only son.

[4] The *bucula* of this stanza is probably distinct from the pregnant *junix* of the last.

[5] "*Pietas*" has a wider sense than English "piety" applying to human as well as divine relations. It overlaps with but has more emotional warmth than English "Duty".

[6] The poetic word *funera* "corpse" tends to humanize the cattle.

109. This sign, placed on the middle of the foreheads of all the herds, was their sure safety. Truly, this is why the god that is powerful in this name is so often called Savior.[7]

113. The severe plague immediately fled away from the herds. The diseases were not permitted to do anything. But nevertheless, if you want to call upon this god (for protection), belief is sufficient. Faith alone helps the prayer.[8]

117. The altar is not wet with any blood, nor is the cattle disease repelled by means of slaughter, but simple purification of the soul attains the good hoped for.

121. Buculus: If you vouch for these things as true, Tityrus, I will make no delay, but I will serve the true sacred ways and gladly flee from the old error, for it is empty and deceitful.

125. Tityrus: But indeed, my mind already hastens to visit the temples of the Supreme God. So come, Buculus; shall we walk a short road together and come to know the divinity of Christ?

129. Aegon: Include me also in your prosperous plans. For why should I doubt that the same sign that conquers the power of disease should not also be of benefit to human beings in the age without end?

End of Severus's Bucolic.

[7] *Salus* "safety", "health" is the base of the word *salvator* "savior", "healer".

[8] For Weitzius, belief "credere" and faith "fides" are synonymous. The poem actually uses the phrase "sola fides" here, "faith alone", which Weitzius adduces in support of the contemporary Lutheran theological position in the note on line 116 below. However, credere and fides are not necessarily synonymous for the original author of the poem since fides in classical Latin can refer more to broader concepts of loyalty and faithfulness.

Notes to this Song, with M. Wolfgang's Seber's Gleanings for this Song

Severus:[1] Gyraldus, citing Sophronius, makes mention of an Attilius or Caecilius Severus, a Christian poet in the reign of the emperor Valentinian (*On Poets, Historical Dialogues,* 5, folio 212). But our man here, it seems, is earlier, and, unless I am greatly mistaken, is from Aquitaine. We owe his song to the benefaction of Élie Vinet of Saintes, a wonderful and very learned old man. This is noted down in Antoine Blanc's 1596 edition.

Bucolic Song: On Bucolic Poetry or Drama, see Scaliger *Poetices,* book 3, chapter 99;[2] Jacob Pontanus's *Poetic Institutes,* book 2, chapter 23; The Giessen *Poetica* book 2, chapter 10.[3]

Deaths: This word is used in the plural number both in Greek and in Latin. See Homer, *Odyssey* 12.341: "*all deaths are hateful.*" Achilles Tatius on the *Love of Clitophorus and Leucippe,* book 4: "*So many are the paths of deaths*"; Plato in the ninth book of the *Laws*: "*to encounter many deaths*" and "*they kill them with deaths*"; Cicero in book 2 of *On Ends*: "the deaths of generals are very glorious"; Seneca in book 1 of *On Clemency, chapter 18*: "O man worthy of a thousand deaths!" And in chapter 1 of *Inquiries on Nature:* "So that you would think that the gods send signs before deaths"; Tacitus, *Histories,* book 3: "By all kinds of deaths"; Virgil Aeneid

[1] The first few notes explain words in the title. The remainder are numbered by line.

[2] By the elder Scaliger.

[3] By the professors of Giessen University.

L. Cole, *The Fifth Plague*, Palgrave Studies in Animals and Literature, https://doi.org/10.1007/978-3-031-92793-5

10.854: "I would have sent my guilty soul through all kinds of deaths"; Lucan, book 7, line 618: "one is ashamed of have spent tears on the funeral of the world with innumerable deaths"; Justinian, *Novella* 85: "Wishing to free human beings from deaths of this type" and 1.17 of the section on betrothals in the *Digests*: "deaths of parents";[4] Latinius Pacatus Drepanius's *Panegyric:* "Am I speaking of the deaths of men?" And again: "who offered their chests to deaths";[5] Salisbury, book 6, chapter 3: "And each one boasted that a thousand deaths had wandered past their heads";[6] Petronius, *Satyricon*: "groins now cold with a thousand deaths"; Martial, book 1, epigram 100: "Four deaths," and book 3, epigram 93: "You rejoice to marry after two hundred deaths," book 6, epigram 33: "deaths of slaves" and again, book 3, epigram 64: "flattering/pleasant deaths," and book 9, epigram 104: "[s/he] forbade that the fertile hydra be repaired by deaths"; Gunther, book 10, line 341: "deaths receive their foundation from all the ether"; Prudentius, 2nd letter against Symmachus: "You, forbid the deaths of wretched men to be consecrated"; but Corinna warned Pindar that one should sow seed with the hand, not by the sackful.

Aegon: *goatherd, driver of goats, goatherd,* goatherd, GOATHERD. Siber in *Gemma* page 441, Petrus Nannius on Virgil's Eclogue 3.[7]

Buculus: *cowherd, leader of the herd;* herdsman, pastor of the herd, COWHERD. Siber. Ibid. and *Gloss.*

Tityrus: for Servius he is "the lead ram."[8] For the earliest Aeolians, it meant "she-goat." Scaliger *On Poetry*, book 1, chapter 12. It may be seen in Becmann's *On Origins*, page 500; Turnebus book 16, chapter 15.[9]

Line 2. "with heavily cast down eyes." Lusininus Euphormio says in the satire:[10] "Of all the parts of the human being, the eyes harmonize with hidden feelings the most, and only strong and lively spirits [or winds] nourish an ample and vigourous gaze. An agreeable one is rather seductive; it indicates that they are easy and not hostile to all pleasures. Likewise, a narrowed eye that flees down into the lowest prison betrays a soul that never rises up by sublime counsels and great thoughts. However, when

[4] *Novels*, Chapter 1, *Digests*, 2.1.17.

[5] One of the twelve Latin Panegyrics, 2.29.1, 2.30.5.

[6] literally "temples" the vulnerable part of the skull. *Policraticus,* 6.594d.

[7] Adam Theodore Siber's *Gemma Gemmarum, or Gem of Gems*, a book on nomenclature with a 1610 edition. Nannius wrote a commentary on Virgil's *Bucolica.*

[8] a late antique commentator on Virgil.

[9] Sixteenth century French Philologist. **Tityros is Doric dialect for Satyros, "Satyr".**

[10] Written by John Barclay.

some disturbance mixes the thunderstruck winds [spirits] of the head so that they can barely sustain the bonds and joints of all the members, the nerves—which descend transversely from the depths of the head into the eyes—especially suffer from the nearby disorder. At that time the nerves depict the hidden disease of the soul through the rapidly trembling eyes and the livid and harsh countenance." And truly Achilles Tatius in book 6 of *on the Love of Clitophon & Leucippe: "I think people who have said that the mind is invisible are completely wrong. For it clearly appears in the face as in a mirror. For when it is pleased, it shines out an image of joy with the eyes, and when in pain, it contracts the face at the sight of the calamity."*[11] Nazarius's Panegyric for Emperor Constantine is also relevant: "An indiscreet pain gave itself away, and it did not fear being perceived; the signs of grief were shut away poorly and expressed themselves through the face." Moreover, lowering the eyes in sadness and grief is more or less in accordance with nature. Euripides's Medea: *"Neither lifting up her eyes, nor removing her face from the ground."* Examples of either type are easy to find.

Line 4. "Let one who loves you know." Aptly, Achilles Tatius in Book 3 of the *Clitophon & Leucippe* says: *"Somehow human beings are affected by the feeling of pity and listen to others' troubles. And pity often furnishes friendship. For the soul is softened towards those whose sorrows it has heard, and by listening to suffering it gradually forms compassion and gathers its pity for sorrow into friendship."*[12] And again in book 6: "*For by nature there is a tear that brings those who see it to pity.*"[13] Euripides harmonizes with this sentiment at *Iphigeneia at Aulis,* line 424: *"It is necessary that friends feel pain in common with friends."* "For affliction is the true bond of friendship, and true friends are proven in the time of adversity, for then the affections are driven to help the friend" according to Book 4, narration 2, page 47 of the *Histories* of P. Matthaeus a royal vernacular author, who is very select and erudite (as Rudolph Botoreus, a man of the same calibur, proclaims in book 16, page 546). Meanwhile, "there is no human being who would wish to adopt the pains and complaints of others as his/her own" acc to Matthaeus in book 2, narration 3, page 203.[14]

[11] 6.6.2.
[12] 3.14.
[13] 6.7.
[14] Line 408.

Line 7. "The one who publishes misfortunes opens a wound." Sedulius in book three, line 416 of the *Paschal Works:* "It is a great medicine to confess that which harms when hidden. For one who covers the plague and fears to bare it to the doctor, nourishes his own wounds." Boethius in book 1, prose section 4: "If you expect help from a doctor, it helps to uncover your wound."

Line 10. "A shared burden becomes lighter." "As labor when shared with many becomes lighter so too does sadness," Lipsius. 2. *De Constantia*, book 2, chapter 26. "Many hands make light work," Erasmus's *Adagia*.

Line 11. "and whatever is covered... more violently." Seneca, *Agamemnon*, line 665: "Cares burn those more whom they lacerate in secret." Ovid *Tristia* 5.1. "A pain that is enclosed chokes and seethes within. It is forced to multiply its strength."

Line 12. "Conversation helps pain." "It is something to be able to lighten a fatal evil by means of talk," says the poet of Sulmo in the *Tristia* 5.1.[15] Aristaenetus agrees with him: *Anyone whose soul is pained on any account, lightens the burden on their mind by calling forth their own grief.*[16] Chrysostom's 5th homily *On the Incomprehensible Nature of God*[17] is of the same mind: "If it brings some consolation to narrate one's calamities and tell of one's misfortunes to other human beings as if the evils were swept away by the act of narration itself, then you will receive a far greater consolation and healing when you communicate the illnesses of your soul to our common Lord." With equal refinement Isidore of Pelusium in book 4, epistle 110: "*For those who cry out and show their suffering to their neighbors, receive no small consolation for their suffering.*"[18] Heliodorus equals these thoughts in book 4: "Take courage and speak. Do not increase sorrow for one in distress by being silent. For any suffering that is quickly known can be helped. But if there is delay in revealing it, then it becomes almost incurable, for silence nourishes diseases, but that which has been drawn out into speech is is easily consoled."[19][...]

Line 18. "The result of the long labor." Horace: "Life gave nothing to mortals without great labor." Phocylides: "*for men, there is no favorable work without labor.*"[20] Pindar in Pythian 12: "*if there is any happiness among*

[15] Ovid.

[16] Epistle 16.

[17] Περὶ τοῦ 'Ακαταλήπτου quoted in Latin translation.

[18] Epistle 1345, line 14.

[19] Heliodorus' *Aethiopica* 4.5.

[20] Line 162. Now considered by Pseudo-Phocylides.

human beings, it does not appear without labor."[21] Timandrides the Spartan returned home after a long journey and found his family property greatly increased. This disturbed him immensely and he said: "O son, the only way this could have happened is that you have injured the majority of gods, family members and guests by your avarice." From Aelian book 14. Clearly he understood that one needs a *long time* if one wishes to gather wealth without the use of force or fraud or evil arts. See Pietro Crinito, *De Honesta Disciplina* book 2, chapter 3 on Furius Cresinus, from Pliny, book 18, chapter 6.

Line 19. "Perished in two days." Euripides's *Phoenician Women*: "*Yet prosperity is not stable but ephemeral.*"[22] For this reason they say (in the fables) that the god of wealth is halt and stumbling when he approaches, but when he departs he does so on the swiftest feet. Cf. Boethius, book 2, prose section 2 and note the harmonies here:

> IN HUMAN LIFE COURAGE AND FORTUNE
> FAIL SUDDENLY FROM BEHIND
> LIKE A WATER-BUBBLE IN THE RAIN
> AND CHANGE LIKE A WEATHERVANE
> From Rolnhag on the *Battle of the Frogs and Mice*, book 1, chapter 6.
> They say: "Wealth has the habit of being halt in his approach, but winged in departure, blind, lacking in judgement."

Line 20. "So quick is the path for evil things!". Symmachus in book 1, epistle 48: "We are born such that we find ourselves more often in adversity. Pleasures flee away and the enjoyment of each good thing is as brief as its perception is fleeting." And rightly Dousa in song 2 of his second book of *Epodes*, based on Plautus Amphitrio [633–635]: "It has little enough of delight in it, little enough of Pleasure. Life is to be lived before bitter things fall upon us. This is what the order of the stars ordains. So it has been found that in this *chaos* Pleasure is followed by greater sorrow as by a kind of companion."[23]

Dominique Baudier, a man of lofty and profound genius has ingeniously said in Iambic Maxims, book 2, chapter 18:[24]

[21] 12.28–29.

[22] Line 558.

[23] Janus Dousa van Noortwiick, "Ad Hadrianum Iunium", in *Libri II Epodon ex Puris Iambis*.

[24] gnom. iamb. or *Gnomae Iambicae*.

Nature proposed a law for prosperity,
that nothing should be perfect in all its parts
lawless pleasure brings penitence
in its train, while grief wounds the flank of joy.

Or as he says with utmost refinement in the same place, section 3:

Life and mortals' lot has these vicissitudes:
that illness be the companion of pleasure;
that hope with fear and fear with hope be tempered
Thus no part of life is free of trouble,
It is decreed that no one can draw from the well of life
water free from these taints. Fortune never brought
any mortal's chariot from the starting stall
as far as the finish without a crash.
IT SO HAPPENS IN THE WORLD
THAT MISFORTUNE DOES STAND BEHIND FORTUNE
GAIN AND LOSS, JOY AND SORROW
ARE VERY CLOSELY RELATED NEIGHBORS
ONE REIGNS OVER THE OTHER
ANYONE WHO CANNOT BEAR IT, SHOULD LEAVE.
And likewise: A sacred grove grows for an uncounted age;
In an instant it perishes from a blast of eager fire.
Our bodies grow with slow vigor.
Suddenly they begin to fail. The slow marching lines of the virtues
are crushed at once; they do not come to life again quickly.

which was written in with acuity in *Wisdom Iambs*, section 32 by Joseph Scaliger, the prince of the erudite, the dictator and parent of letters, the greatest work of nature and a marvel while he lived.[25]

Line 21. "dire plague." Ovid, *Metamorphoses* 7.523: "A dire plague fell upon the peoples." [...] Prudentius, *Hamartigenia*, line 861: "Which dire plague and malignant error immersed in darkness."

Line 21. "creep." Ammianus Marcellinus, book 19: "That destruction gradually crept forth from as far as the boiling clime of Ethiopia."[26] Lucretius, book 6, line 1120: "and even the unfriendly air began to creep." Virgil, 3rd *Georgic*, line 369: Dire contagions creep through the unwary

[25] *Iambi Gnomici.*

[26] 19.4.4. He compares Thucydides' plague with a contemporary one.

common people. Prudentius, in first *Book against Symmachus*, line 538: "creeping poison."

Line 22. "long ago." Nay, "there is no nation under the sun that does not have complaints and oppressions" as is said by P. Matthaeus, a man of ingenious discernment and deep erudition in book 2, page 197, of his *Histories.* "And somehow or other this pestilential Madness walks abroad in this world with a swifter foot than pure Prayers do," Lipsius, *Miscellanies*, 1st cento, epistle 91.[27] Hence Pindar, *Nemean 7:* "*the wave of Hades comes to all. It falls on those who expect it and upon those who do not.*"[28] "Those things that are born are urged along by their end," according to D. Hilarius, On Genesis, line 22.

Line 33. "strong [bodies of] oxen." Ovid, *Letters from Pontus* 1.5: "You perceive that hard labor in the fields breaks the strong bodies of bull (and what is more enduring than a bovine?)." An ox or a bull has an exceedingly robust and strong nature according to Johann Thomas Freigius, in *Quaestiones Physicae*, book 34, page 1084. Hence Virgil, 1st *Georgic*: "Strong bulls."

Line 38. "the same tameness." Oppian's *Hunting with Dogs*, 2.88: "thinking tame thoughts, accustomed to (speaking) human beings." Lucretius, 3.303: "But the nature of bovines lives better with calm air. Nor is it stirred up by the smoky torch of excessive anger pouring out shadows of blind darkness below." Or does Ovid call those tame "whom the use of the plow helps? For Bullocks refuse the yoke when first seized." Amores 1.2.

Line 51. "shaking with long spasms in his flanks" Virgil, *3rd Georgic*, line 505:

> "But then the eyes burn and the deeply drawn breath is drawn deeply, sometimes with a heavy groan while the flanks are tense with long sobs."[...]

Line 54. "By your losses just as by my own." For as Prudentius sings:

> "The same law warns all
> to groan beneath the same lot" (*Cathemerinon* 10)
> and "Anything that can happen to anyone can happen to *anyone.*"
> Callion understood this when he was composing a letter in the presence of Euphormio Lusininus to his friend Fibullius who was sick with a kidney stone on page 42 of the *Satyricon* and used these words: "That the breath of

[27] Madness and prayers are personified. Lipsius' *Epistolarum Selectarum Centuria Prima Miscellanea*.

[28] A second meaning: "upon those who are famous and those who are not". *Nemean* 7.31.

> those who love is drawn from another's mouth is not so much something that I learned from the example of others. Rather I myself can be an example of this. As long as you were in perfect health I lived in you. When your health was afflicted, my pain was greater [than yours], since the sickness of your body wounded my mind" and so on. See page 190 of the same book.[29]

Line 63 "souls." "Anima" is used for the life of brutes that vanishes with them and returns to nothing. [...]

Line 72. "drew the plague from her udder." For "all things look back to their origin," as Salvian says in book 6 of *On the Governance*. [...] "That which comes from filth, what can it become but filth? For 'it is not possible for a bad tree to produce good fruit' since the force of nature resides in it so that like is produced from like." Salisbury, book 5. chapter 11.[30]

Line 75. "lowing." Valerius Flaccus, book 8, line 457: For cows to draw sighing breaths. Likewise Claudian in book 1, line 128 of the *De Raptu Proserpinae* on the love of a cow for her offspring: "No more mildly does the stern parent circle her calf who has not yet crossed the field on its feet. Nor has its forehead received the crescent curves of new horns." To this add Lucretius 2.352. Oppian's *Halieutica* 1.724, and *Cynegetica* 3.107 ff.[31] Quintus Smyrnaeus 7.254, where Deidamia weeping at the departure of Neoptolemus is compared with a cow seeking her lost calf. The same author compares Andromache to a cow as well at 13.258: "*But she bewails her dear offspring to the goddess and laments loudly hither and thither.*"[32]

Line 76. "and wished to die." Behold the "*physical affection towards their children*" even in brutes and be astounded by it! Diodorus has choice words on this theme in book 2 of the *Bibliotheca Historica* "*Nature is good at teaching all living things to preserve, not only themselves but also those that are born from them. It does this through the inborn love of life which leads the generations into an eternal cycle of perpetuation.*"[33]

Line 84. "collapses." Thus Nemesis *punishes* wantonness even in brutes.

Line 85. "As many falling leaves from a forest." *Aeneid* 6.309: "As many as the leaves that slip and fall in the first frost of Autumn." The

[29] The *Euphormionis Lusinini Satyricon*, a picaresque novel by John Barclay.

[30] *Policraticus*.

[31] The *Halieutica* is a five-book second century didactic epic on fishing. *The Cynegetica* is often considered the slightly later work of a different anonymous author.

[32] 13.254–262.

[33] 2.50.7.

opposite is found in Valerius Flaccus 6.167: "With so many leaves, with so many flowers does the year begin." Compare Seneca in line 600 of the *Oedipus;* Zehner Biblical Similitudes, chapter 101. Virgil's 3rd *Georgic* uses a *simile* of this kind at line 600:

> "Not so many the storms that rush upon the main in advance of winter
> as the multitude of plagues of cattle."
> Ovid, *Metamorphoses* 7.585 expresses the matter in such a way:
> "The populace was laid low like rotting fruit fallen
> from the shaken boughs, like acorns cast off from the oak."

Line 93. "of sad ill-omened birds" [...] Ammianus, book 31: "Ill-omened birds consumed the remaining bodies of the slain.[34] At that time they were in the habit of feeding on cadavers as the plains white with bones show even now." [...] Statius in *Thebaid* book 9 names them: "bands of impure birds to whom from far away the breeze brought the noxious air and abandoned deaths lacking funerals."[35]

Line 102. "What god snatched you out of these calamities?" One should only assign it to God Optimus Maximus[36] when we are delivered out of a crisis or freed from evil. "*There is nothing that god cannot do*" according to the Pythagorean Epicharmus as quoted in Clement of Alexandria's *Stromateis.*[37] "*Nothing can stand against his will,*" Bardisanes the Syrian, from Eusebius book 6.[38] "*[God] found a solution for the unexpected,*" Euripides.[39] See Hadrianus Junius, proverb 1, from cento 8: "When God goes before, no obstacle stands in the way."[40]

Line 107. "Christ, the glory of the Divinity." Taken without doubt from Hebrews 1.3, in which passage Christ is named "*radiance of the glory and impress of the hypostasis of God.*" But δόξα (*doxa*), which we commonly translate as "gloria," sometimes indicates the divine and heavenly radiance of light and splendor, as one may see at Exodus 34.30 on the effulgence

[34] 31.7.16.

[35] 9.27–29.

[36] "Best and Highest", old Roman epithets for Jupiter, used by Christian authors in the Renaissance.

[37] 5.14.100. This is also quoted in Eusebius' *Praeparatio Evangelica*, 13.13.25, though not noted by our author.

[38] 6.10.48.

[39] This phrase appears five times in Euripides' plays: *Bacchae* v. 1391; *Helen* v. 1691; *Andromache* v. 1287; *Medea* v. 1418; *Alcestis* v. 1162!

[40] Presumably proverb 801 from his 850 proverb supplement to Erasmus' *Adagia*.

of Moses's face, and 2nd Corinthians 3.7, Luke 2.9. ἀπαύγασμα, however, denotes the shining that is reflected from that radiance. Therefore, just as light is known from its (reflected) shining, and as the weak eyes of mortals more readily bear the reflected shining of the sun than the direct rays of the solar body, just so the Son is indicated as the reflected shining and emanation of that eternal glory and radiance in God, D. G. Myl. in the passage on the Person of Christ.

Line 109. "added to the middle of the foreheads." Thus Prudentius in the *Cathemerinon*, book 6, line 129:

> "When sleep calls and you seek your chaste bed,
> See that the sign of the cross seals the forehead and the place of the heart...etc"
> See the following passages of the same work and on Romanus, line 586 and 621.[41] Alfonsus Ciacco wrote about the sign of the Cross.[42]

Line 115. "Belief is sufficient." *"Just have trust."* Mark 5.36, Luke 9.50.

Line 116. "Faith alone." The Papists hate the excluding particle *"like the gates of Hades."*[43] Nevertheless Orthodox fathers, both Greek and Latin have used it. On this matter, see Dr. Lobechius's 7th *Disputation on the Articles of the Augsburg Confession on page 154 and the following page; Dr. Hutter's explanation of the Formula of Concord pa*ge 321 and the following pages.[44]

Line 119. "But simple purification of the soul... the hoped for." Lactantius *Epitome* of the *Divine Institutes,* chapter 2: "Therefore, what does GOD want from human beings except cultiviation of the mind which is pure and holy? For those things which are made by the fingers or are outside of the human being, this is not a true sacrifice, nor that which comes out of a box, but that which is brought forth from the heart, not that libation which is made by hand, but that which is made with the mind. This is an acceptable victim which the soul immolates from itself. For what is the use of sacrifices? What the use of incense? What of vestments? Of gold? Of silver? What good do precious stones do if the mind

[41] *Cathemerinon* or "Poem that Follows the Hours of the Day". "Romanus" refers to a section of Prudentius' *Peristephanon* "On the crowns of the martyrs".

[42] Probably Alphonsus Ciacconius (1530–1599).

[43] Probably a paraphrase of Achilles words in Iliad 9.312, in which he hates a liar like the gates of death. Spoken to the famous liar Odysseus.

[44] David Lobechius and Leonhard Hutter were Lutheran scholars.

of the worshiper is not pure?" See book 6, chapters 24 and 25 of the same work. Marcus Minucius Felix's *Octavius*: "Shall I offer hosts and victims to the Lord, which he gave me for my use, so that I would cast back his own gift to him? It is ungrateful, since a fit offering would be a good soul and a pure mind and an honest conscience..." and so on. The Divine Bernard in his *Sententiae*: "For us to be reconciled to GOD, we do not need works or signs, but purity and simplicity of heart..." and so on.

Line 124. "for it is deceitful." Lactantius said it very well in book 4, chapter 3: "Therefore truth cannot be grasped when the same human being is subject to many fathers and masters, when the soul is dispersed in many things and wanders hither and thither and is unable to have any firmness, when religion lacks a certain and stable home. Therefore the cults of the gods cannot be true, in the same way that it cannot be called marriage when one woman has many men, but she is called either a prostitute or an adulteress. For she who is far from modesty, purity and faithfulness must necessarily lack virtue. Thus the religion of the gods is also immodest and uncertain, because it lacks faithfulness, since an unstable and uncertain honor has no head or origin."

Line 129. "Include me also in your prosperous plans." This is the same advice that wise Cato used to give: "Walk with good people." Hence the Divine Ambrose in book 2 of *On the Calling of the Nations* at the end of chapter 10: "While they have life in this body, no one's correction should be neglected; no one's repair should be despaired of."[45]

> And these are the observations and notes that I was permitted to make on this very elegant ode. My comments are not to be numbered among gems or the wares of the Indies
> but should be reckoned cheaper than the pebbles or seaweed of the shore.
> Therefore I set no price to them, but scatter them out like public alms.

M. Wolfgang
Seber's Gleanings
for this Song

Line 2. "Cast down." Scholion on Euripides's *Orestes*, line 253 (Where Electra says *"Woe is me, brother, your eye is troubled!"): "In accordance with nature, for the eyes are images of all the passions of the soul."* The Publican in

[45] Scholars now debate whether Ambrose or Prosper of Aquitaine wrote *De Vocatione Omnium Gentium*.

Luke 18.13 would be an especially good example: *"Neither gazing at wide heaven, the throne of the great God, but staring down at the pavement with servile eyes,"* from Gregory Nazianzus's *Song on his own Life*, line 402.

Line 5. "I beg you let me... in deep...." Similarly Ovid in Tristia book 4.4.40: "But allow me not to remember my fate and do not break open wounds that have not yet cohered by handling them again; rest itself will barely help them."

Proverb: "Do not stir up an evil that has been buried." From line 423 of Theognis.

Line 11. "Whatever is covered." Justin's *Histories*, book 8 (page 103 in my version): "Grief increases for very dissimulation; the less he is allowed to admit it, the more deeply depressed he becomes." And the most learned Panhypersebasta, the daughter of the great Logothete speaks of this at greater length in book 8 of Nicephorus Gregoras *Histories* on folio 139:[46] *"As olive oil, wax, reeds and grass are the natural food of fire, just so when silence finds the coals of grief ready around the soul it gives itself to them as nourishment (f. luxury) and food, and it does not move aside (L. allow) for the smoke that builds up in the soul to escape."* And shortly after that passage: *"In a way, terrible grief most easily multiplies when there is extended silence"* and so on.[47]

Line 27. "Why did you not prevent it in advance." Compare this with Theognis 1130: *"Let us seek medicines for a swelling sore."* Similar examples can be found everywhere.

Line 29. "No obvious signs of this fearsome thing." It seems that Thucydides described the plague of Attica seizing people in a similar way: "*from no cause, but suddenly.*" "No clear or manifest cause appeared, but [it came] suddenly." On this passage the scholion writer noted: "*without apparent cause.*" In any case, observing and measuring the signs of diseases help greatly in driving them away. Hence one division of Medicine is entitled "Semiotic,"[48] and Herophilus introduced "*tri-temporal observation of symptoms*"[49] which would indicate the signs of a state of health,

[46] These are Byzantine court titles. Gregoras' history is an important source for the fourteenth century.

[47] The parentheses in this note are Seber's. They apparently note textual variants. The change of one letter makes the difference in meaning for the second. A difference in prefix makes for a smaller difference of meaning in the third. The letter abbreviations may refer to specific manuscripts.

[48] Literally: "that which pertains to signs".

[49] *semeiosis trichronos.*

signs which were distinguished by a triple series of times, as handed down from Hippocrates and Galen by Gorrh. in the *Definit.*[50] and by Anutius Foesius in his *Lexicon Hippocraticum.* In this same vein it seems that Buculus, even though he is only talking about his own herd animals, complains that the disease is so virulent that the animals catch it and die simultaneously, while no obvious indications appear. That is, there were no signs that would show one that there was any opportunity for using the medical art, so that the signs would be obvious, clear, manifest, and such that can be understood by intellect.

Line 35. "twin mind." It is my opinion that mind has been used for sound. For it happens that through sound rattles and chimes and bells seem to live and all but have minds especially if a number of them sound together in sweet harmony and express the melody of definite songs. This artifice is not completely unknown to our own people; however, much foreigners may have boasted about it up to this point. See Girolamo Maggi's *On Bells*, chapter 17, with the notes of Franciscus Sweertius.

Line 38. "Tameness." Patience. On this, Ovid, *Tristia* 5.4 "With time, the bull becomes patient with the rustic plow." For Propertius attests to this in book 2, elegy 3: "At first the bull refuses the plow. Afterwards he comes to the field broken in to the familiar yoke." And thence in line 46: "The second summer that had seen him tamed."

Line 63. "Young heifer." Lucius Annaeus Cornutus, commenting on Persius's 2nd Satire says: "Young heifers [iunices] are said to be bovines of tender years who have just ceased to be calves but have not yet reached their full size."

Line 90. "swell with bulging." This happens at times, if not always, to bodies that have been seized by poison taken in with the feed. As Pliny writes: "the cattle burst after devouring *buprestis.*"[51] This insect is similar to the long-footed beetle.[52] It often encounters cattle unobserved in the grass.

Line 93. "Sad ill-omened birds." Sad and ill-omened birds which in Iliad 1.4 are called *"Birds."* Shorter Scholion: *"Flesh-eating birds,"* "carnivorous birds" as are vultures and ravens. Plutarch, *Sympotic Questions* 8.9:[53] "Thucydides records that the plague at Athens was unusual. He judged its unusualness especially from the fact that scavenging animals did

[50] Probably *Definitiones.*

[51] Buprestis is the name of a kind of vegetable but also of a beetle with a venemous sting.

[52] *scarabaeus longipes.*

[53] 733 B.2 in modern editions.

not touch the dead." The passage in Thucydides is from book 2, folio 131, W.[54]

Line 98. "Leapt across some." Something of this sort happened long ago in Egypt when the Lord sent a great plague on the domestic animals through Moses; since meanwhile not one of the Israelites animals died, Exodus 9.3–6.

Line 102. "god." Synesius, epistle 139: "*When god is present, every impossibility is possible.*"

Line 107. "Christ the glory of the Divinity." Philippians 2.11: "Let every tongue confess *that Christ Jesus is Lord to the glory of god the father.*"

Line 109. "This sign added to the foreheads of the herds was their safety." On the sign or figure of the Cross: if a human being should sign himself with it with true faith in Christ crucified, let it be so. Athanasius's *Oratio contra Gentes section. 1, folio 1: "Every phantasy of the demons is driven away by this sign." On the Incarnation of the Word,* in the same volume, folio 61: "*At the sign of the cross every magic ceases, every sorcerous drug is rendered null.*" See folio 75, of the same volume. But I said, "*if* with *true* faith in Christ crucified."[55] For in his *Vita* by Athanasius, *according to page 17 of the cleric Haeschelius' recent edition based on a* handwritten codex, Anthony says: "*For we have one seal and wall for security: our faith in the Lord.*"[56] Haeschelius has an old [Latin] translation elsewhere in volume 2, folio 447: "the sign of the Cross and an unconquerable faith in the Lord are a defensive wall for us." But without faith, it is dangerous to make the form of the Cross by itself nor is it at all safe for a human being, as the object of the following inauspicious song found out: "Sign signs for yourself! Touch me without respect and feel pain."[57] Yet what about the sign of the Cross for cows and other brute animals? *Does God really care about cows?* [1st Cor. 9.9] One could fittingly apply 1st Corinthians 9.9 to this. It is pure superstition involving great impiety to derive the salvation of bovines or domestic animals from the decree of redemption. This is said in Psalm 36.7: "You will save beasts of burden, O Lord." This is only to be accepted concerning providence and preservation. Psalm 104.14, 147.9, Matthew 6.26, etc. also pertain to this.

[54] W. probably indicates a specific edition. 2.47–55 in modern texts.

[55] My italics here express words emphasized in Latin.

[56] 9.40.

[57] The jingling Latin also evokes the "do not touch me" addressed to Mary Magdalene.

Line 116. "Faith alone." The word "alone" is a thorn in papal eyes.[58] But it is supported by the evident testimony of both Scripture itself and of the learned and divine Fathers. The cleric Zehner produces a long list of such Fathers in his *Compendium Theologiae* page 474 and the following.[59]

Line 122. "I will serve true." Cyprian, in the *Sentences of the Bishops, Decree 30, Folio 447:* "after truth has been revealed, let custom yield to truth."

[58] This combines the speck and beam imagery of Matthew 7.3–5 with Paul's thorn in the flesh.

[59] Probably Joachim Zehner, a Lutheran cleric and scholar who lived from 1566–1612 and appears to have written three different *Compendia Theologiae*.

Index[1]

[1] Note: Page numbers followed by 'n' refer to notes.

L. Cole, *The Fifth Plague*, Palgrave Studies in Animals and Literature, https://doi.org/10.1007/978-3-031-92793-5

D

Q

FSC
www.fsc.org
MIX
Papier | Fördert
gute Waldnutzung
FSC® C083411

Kolibri 360 GmbH
Ferdinand-Jühlke-Straße 7
99095 Erfurt, Deutschland
produktsicherheit@kolibri360.de